P9-CED-416

Carolyn Taylor's

Home Haircuts and Styles

For Men And Boys

Developed by
CAROLYN TAYLOR

Special Consultant
WILLIAM A. ANDERSON

Written by
GARY HOGG

Copyright © 1989 by Anderson Publishing Company and
Carolyn Taylor.

All rights reserved. Published in the United States by
Anderson Publishing Company.

Reproducing all or part of this book in any form without
the written permission of Anderson Publishing or
Carolyn Taylor is strictly prohibited.

INTRODUCTION

After over 25 years of cutting hair, I still find it very rewarding to see the satisfied smiles on the faces of those whose hair I cut. It's a wonderful feeling. It's a feeling that you also will experience as you master the techniques described in this book and give professional looking haircuts to your family and friends within the confines of your home.

The process of cutting hair may seem complicated to you. However, when a haircut is broken down into small, easy-to-follow steps, it is greatly simplified. Each of these steps is thoroughly explained and carefully illustrated in this book. By patiently following the instructions, you will be able to perform any of the haircuts with ease.

Think of anything new that you have learned in your life. It probably took time and effort for you to master the new skill. After practice and patience, you can now execute the task with ease. The same is true for giving a haircut. The first haircut you give will probably take more time than you expect. However, after each haircut, you will find that it becomes faster and easier.

It is best to read completely through the haircut instructions a couple of times in order to get a feel for what you are going to be doing. You may even want to perform a dry run, going through the steps of the haircut, but not actually cutting.

Relax. Don't get in a hurry, and you too will be able to give great looking haircuts.

*I*NDEX

EQUIPMENT

In order to give a professional haircut, you must use professional haircutting equipment. Using inferior equipment, or trying to get by without the proper tools is asking for trouble. You will become frustrated and give a less than satisfactory haircut. Give yourself every advantage by using all of the equipment described in this book. These tools were designed specifically for haircutting and will produce the best results.

Once you have accumulated all of the necessary equipment, put it in a box or bag and label it as your haircutting kit. Doing this will serve two purposes. First, it will keep all of the tools together in one place. This eliminates searching for your tools every time you give a haircut. Second, it will serve as a reminder not to use your haircutting tools for purposes other than haircutting. Using your clamps or scissors for purposes other than hair care is a fast and easy way to ruin their effectiveness.

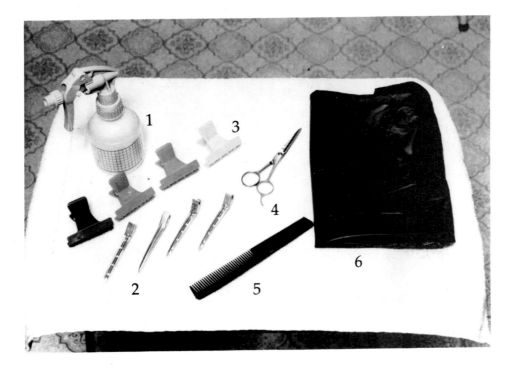

HAIRCUTTING EQUIPMENT NEEDED: **1.** Squirt Bottle **2.** Duckbill Clamps **3.** Butterfly Clamps **4.** Scissors **5.** Comb **6.** Cape.

CHAIR

The most important feature of the stool or chair you use is the height. It should be high enough that you can cut the person's hair without having to bend over. Your back will tire quickly if you bend over for the entire haircut. It is also more difficult to cut the hair evenly when you are bending over. If the chair is not high enough, use books or pillows to raise the person up to the proper height.

It is best if the chair doesn't have any arms. Working around the arms of a chair can be awkward and may impair your ability to cut the hair evenly.

MIRROR

Have the person whose hair you are cutting sit in front of a mirror. At various times, you will need to look in the mirror to ensure that you are cutting the hair evenly. Hand held mirrors are generally too small and should be avoided.

SCISSORS

It is ridiculous to imagine a surgeon performing an operation with a steak knife, instead of a scalpel. While steak knives and scalpels are both cutting instruments, they are obviously designed for different types of cutting. The same is true when it comes to different kinds of scissors.

Sewing and household scissors will not produce a professional looking haircut. You should use only professional hair cutting scissors when giving a haircut.

COMB

The professional styling comb is designed to fit easily and comfortably in your hand. It has big teeth on one end and small teeth on the other. Hair is easier to part off and comb through with this kind of comb.

HAIR CLAMPS

There are two types of clamps used in hair cutting, butterfly and duckbill clamps. They are designed for convenience and holding the hair securely in place. Avoid using bobby pins or other substitutes. They will not hold the hair as well and will tend to cause frustrations.

CAPE

The cape is a great asset in controlling where the hair goes. It will keep the hair off of the clothes of the person whose hair you are cutting and catch the majority of the hair before it reaches the floor. It should be fastened around the neck so that it is snug, yet comfortable.

SQUIRT BOTTLE

During the haircut, it is essential to keep the hair wet. The hair combs smoother and more evenly when it is wet. In order to keep the hair damp throughout the haircut you will need to spray it periodically.

GENERAL INSTRUCTIONS

The first thing to prepare before giving a haircut is yourself. You must place yourself in a positive state of mind. When you have confidence in yourself, the people whose hair you cut will have more confidence in you and your abilities.

Take some time and review the steps of the haircut you are going to give. The more familiar you are with the haircut, the more at ease you will feel when giving it.

Avoid making negative statements about your abilities or the haircut. Making excuses or apologies before or during the cut will condition the person to expect a bad haircut.

Extend every courtesy to the person whose hair you are cutting. Showing respect by being courteous will increase the respect the person will have for you.

The first few times you cut hair, it is important that the person whose hair you are cutting has plenty of patience. If he grows restless, you will be tempted to race through the haircutting process. This will definitely result in a less than satisfactory haircut.

Before giving any haircut, the hair must be properly prepared. This preparation begins with a thorough shampoo. Clean hair is more manageable and cuts more smoothly.

Towel dry the hair, leaving it damp. It is important that the hair remain damp throughout the entire haircut. Wet hair holds together better and allows you to get a much more even cut. Keep a squirt bottle handy to wet the hair when it begins to dry.

Once the hair has been washed and towel dried, you must comb out all of the tangles. When combing through tangled hair, always begin at the bottom and work your way up. Trying to force a comb through tangled hair from the top down will stretch the hair and break off some of the ends.

Every haircut in this book utilizes a systematic approach to cutting hair. First, the hair is sectioned according to the bone structure of the head. This not only makes it easier to cut the hair, but it customizes each haircut for the individual's head shape and size.

For the majority of cuts you make during a haircut, you are holding the hair between your fingers. Always hold the hair snug and straight from the head. Holding the hair loosely or at an awkward angle from the head will result in a less than satisfactory cut.

Once the hair is sectioned off, you will begin cutting. A successful haircut is given in small snips and clips. Cutting a large portion of hair at one time leads to an uneven haircut. Cutting small amounts of hair gives you the control necessary to achieve a professional looking haircut.

The first cut you make in each section will serve as the guide for cutting the rest of the section. This technique allows you to keep the length consistent, producing a smooth, even haircut.

The pictures and text of this book are designed to work together in explaining each procedure. Be sure to study the picture and read the accompanying text before you make any cuts.

THE BASIC HAIRCUT

The basic haircut is the hallmark of men's hairstyles. It is a versatile haircut that allows a person to comb his hair into many different styles.

After you master the techniques of this haircut you will be able to cut hair in many of the fads or styles of the day by using the basic methods described here. Learn this haircut well and it will serve you well for years to come.

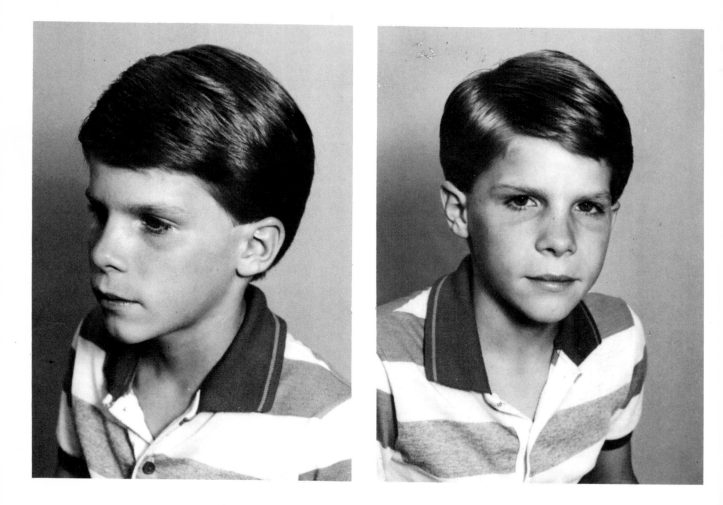

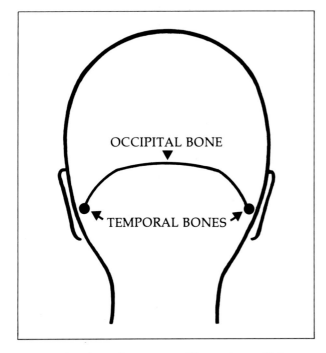

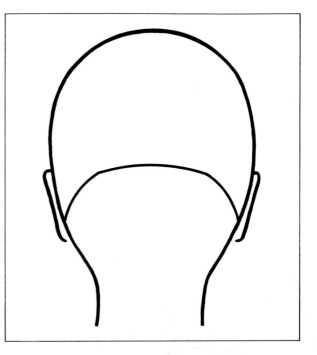

A-1 The first division will section off the *nape* area. The nape area goes from the bottom of the skull down to and including the neck. The bones which will be used to guide the division of this section are the *occipital* and *temporal* bones.

The occipital bone forms the base of the skull. To locate it, slide your fingertips down the back of the skull until you feel where the skull curves in. The large bone you can feel at this point is the occipital bone.

To locate the temporal bone, feel the skull behind one of the ears. Approximately half the distance down the ear you will feel the rounded end of the temporal bone.

A-2 Using the comb, make a part in the hair which runs from one temporal bone up to the occipital bone and down to the other temporal bone. The completed part should look like an arch.

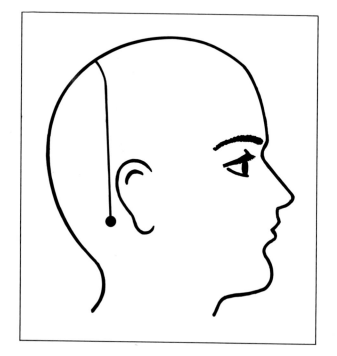

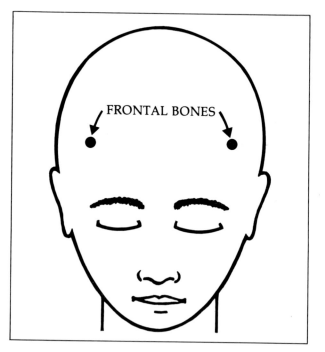

FRONTAL BONES

A-3 The next division will separate the front of the head from the back. From one of the temporal bones, make a part that runs straight up the side of the head to the crown and then down the opposite side to the other temporal bone.

A-4 The next two partings of the hair will establish the dividing lines between the top and sides of the head. To make these divisions, you need to locate the *frontal* bones. The frontal bones are found on both sides of the head at the top of the forehead approximately above the outer end of the eyebrow line.

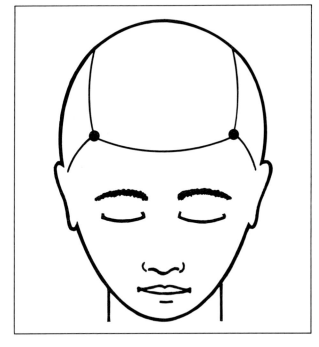

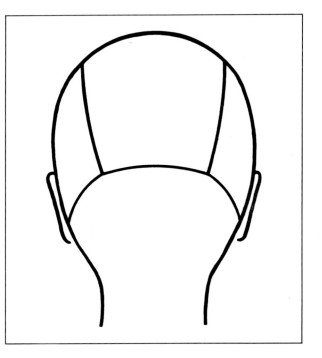

A-5 From each frontal bone, make a part that runs straight back to the part which runs over the crown of the head. Now comb the hair on top of the head which is between the two frontal parts towards the center of the head and clamp in place using a *butterfly* clamp.

A-6 Continue each frontal bone part straight down the back of the head to the nape area part. This will create *three* divisions of the back section of the head. Using butterfly clamps, securely clamp the hair of each division so that it stays in its place.

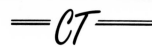

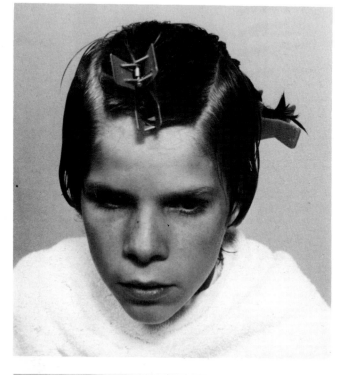

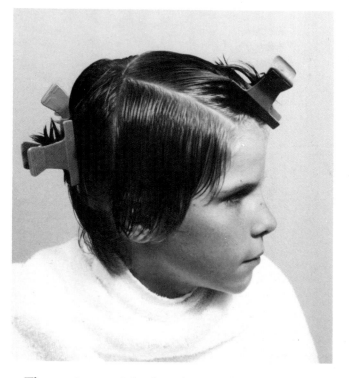

Three views of the head once the hair has been combed into the different sections.

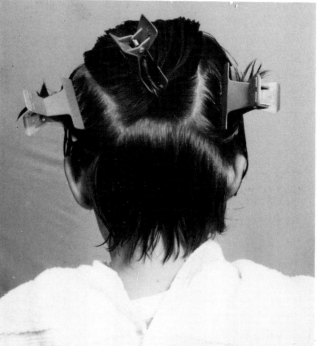

CUTTING THE NAPE AREA

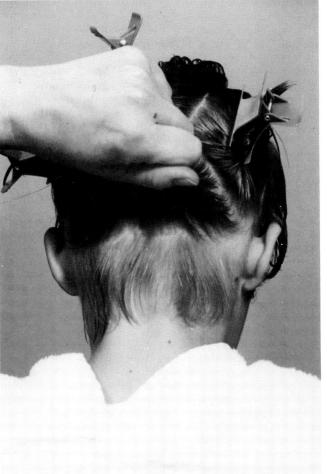

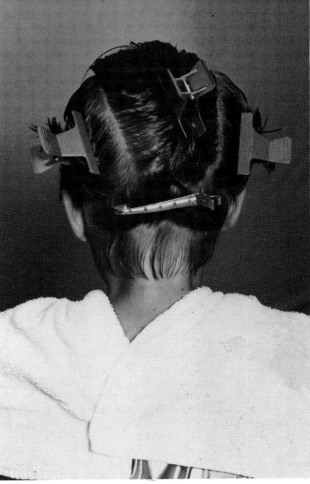

B-1 With the comb, part off the bottom third of the hair of the nape area. Twist and clamp the remaining hair with a *duckbill* clamp.

B-2 Comb the unclamped hair straight down, letting it fall naturally.

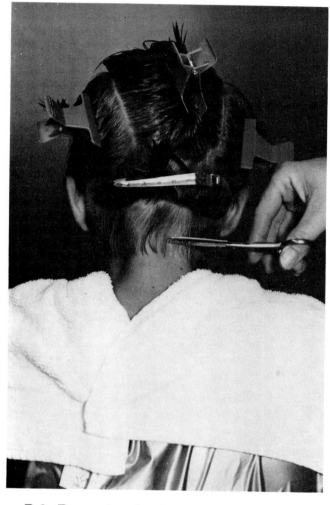

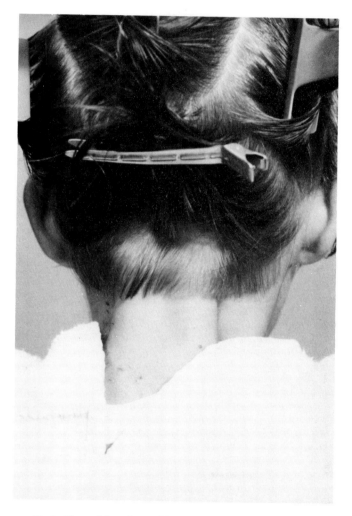

B-3 Determine the desired length and cut the hair straight across, rounding the corners.

B-4 Stand back and look at the hair to make sure that it has been cut straight. This hair will serve as your guide for making the next cut.

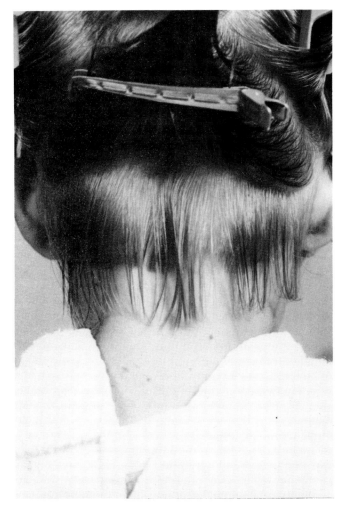

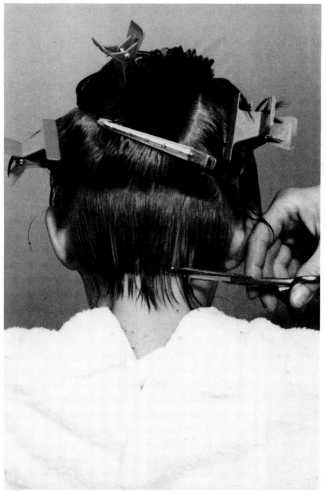

B-5 Remove the duckbill clamp and part off the second third of the nape area hair. If you *can't* see the hair you have already cut through the second third, you have parted off *too much* hair. Reclamp the remaining hair.

B-6 Cut this hair the *exact same length* as the guide hair.

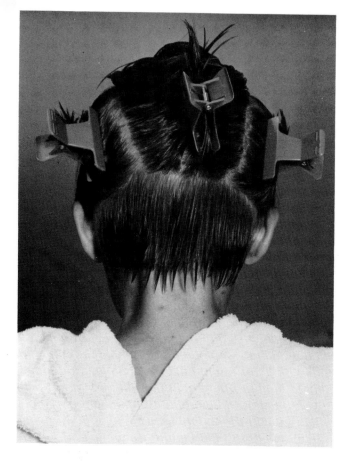

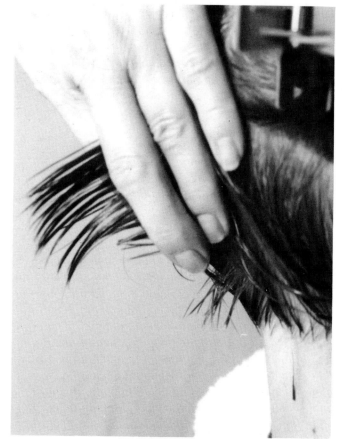

B-7 Remove the duckbill clamp from the remaining hair in the nape area and comb it smoothly down.

B-8 Comb and pick up a vertical section of hair in the middle of the nape area running from the top of the nape area down to and including some of the hair you previously cut. This section should *not* exceed a 1/2 inch in width.

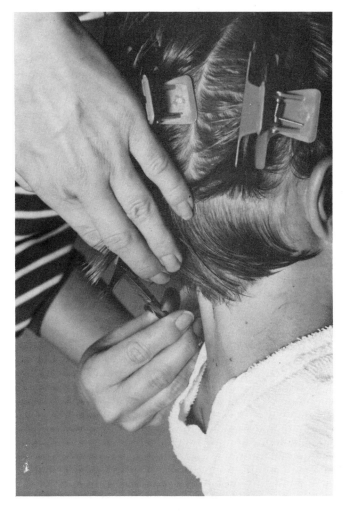

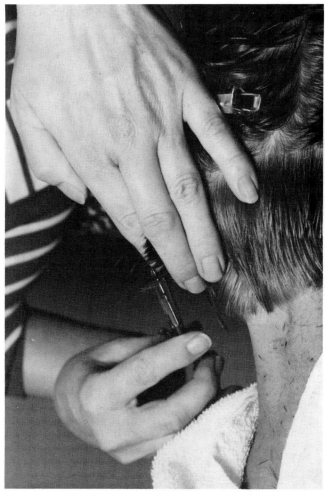

B-9 Using the previously cut hair which is near your fingertips as your guide, cut the hair which is between your fingers.

B-10 Part off another vertical section of hair which is to the left of but includes some of the hair you just cut. Using this previously cut hair as your guide, cut the section you are holding. Continue picking up and cutting sections, using the hair from each previous cut as your guide, until you have cut the entire left half of the nape area.

Repeat this procedure to cut the right side of the nape area.

CUTTING THE BACK

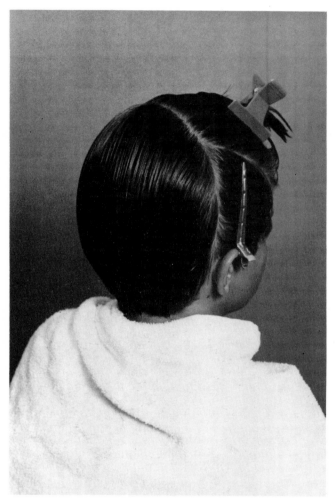

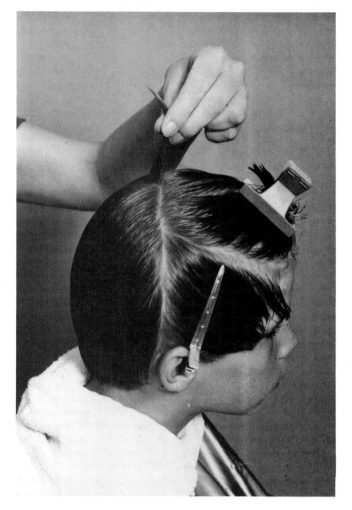

C-1 Comb the hair on the side of the head forward and clamp it into place with a duckbill clamp. Remove the clamps from the back of the head and comb the hair smoothly down.

C-2 At the crown of the head, pick up a ¼ inch section of hair between your thumb and index finger. Run your thumb and index finger, pinched together, up this hair a few times until the hair sticks together. Holding this hair straight up from the head, let go of it and it will fall back to the head, forming an arch.

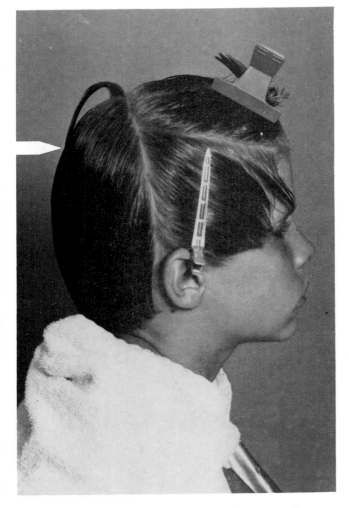

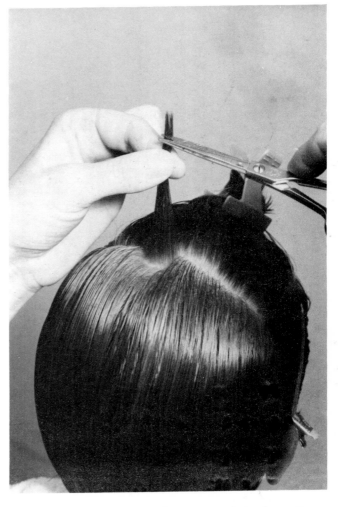

C-3 Take hold of the arch of hair at the *exact* point where it touches the head.

C-4 Cut this hair at the *exact* point where it touched the head. This technique insures that the hair is cut the proper length for the individual.

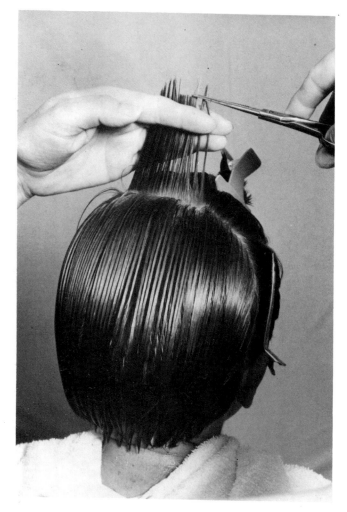

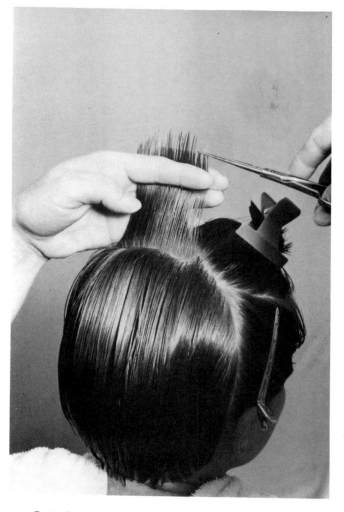

C-5 Comb and pick up a horizontal section of hair, which runs approximately an inch on each side of the arch of hair you just cut. Using the shorter hair in the middle of the section as your guide, cut the hair.

C-6 Just below the hair you just cut, comb and part off another section of hair. Be sure to include some of the hair you just cut in this section to serve as a guide. Cut this section the same length as the guide.

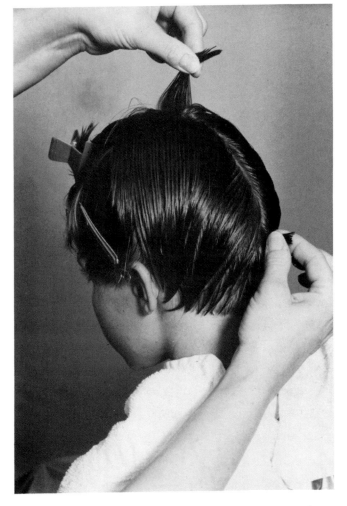

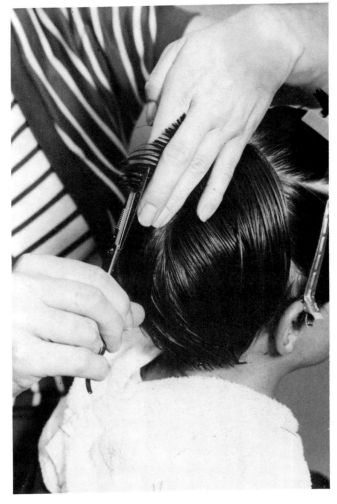

C-7 With your left hand, hold up a piece of crown hair that has been cut. Directly below this hair, with your right hand, pick up a piece of hair from the top of the nape area which has been cut. Holding up these two pieces of hair allows you to easily see the angle the hair needs to be cut in order for the back to blend with the nape area.

C-8 In between the two points, comb and part off a section of hair approximately a ¼ of an inch wide. Be sure to include some of the hair cut from the crown to serve as a guide. Cut this section using the crown hair as a guide.

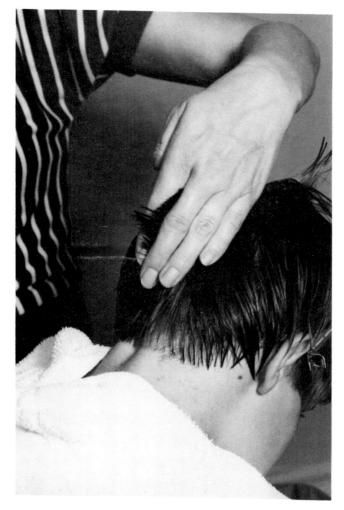

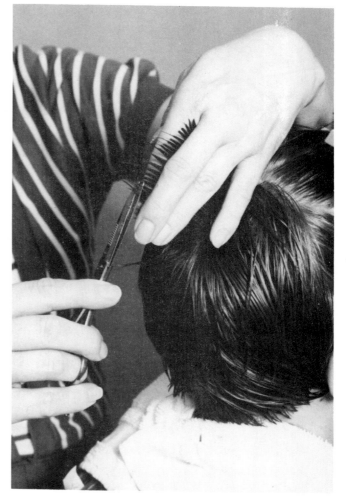

C-9 Comb and part off the next section below the section you just cut. In this section, be sure to include both hair from the section you just cut and hair from the top of the nape area. Cut the hair so that it angles between the two points.

C-10 The vertical section that you just cut will serve as the guide for making the next cut. Beginning at the crown, comb and part off a vertical section to the left of, but including some of the previously cut hair. Use the previously cut hair as a guide and cut this hair. Continue parting off and cutting sections of hair working to the left. *Always use the hair just previously cut as your guide.*

Repeat this procedure working in sections until the right side is cut.

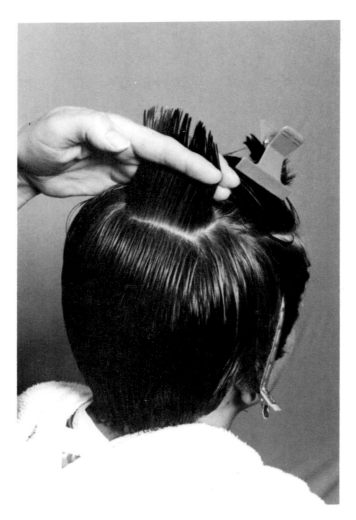

C-11 Recheck the back section by picking up horizontal sections of hair and snipping off any hairs that stick up above the length the rest of the hair is cut. Continue picking up sections until you have checked the entire back.

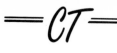

CUTTING THE SIDES

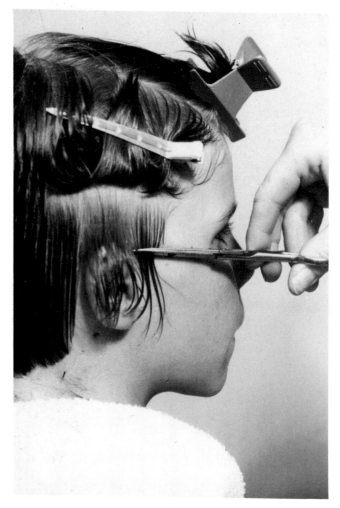

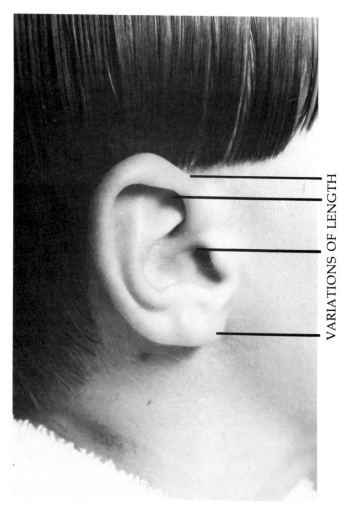

VARIATIONS OF LENGTH

D-1 Remove the duckbill clamp and make a horizontal part in the hair ½ inch above the ear. Reclamp the remaining hair.

D-2 In deciding on the desired length for the side, it is best to have the length coordinate with some part of the ear. By doing this, you will be able to use that part of the ear as a gauge in getting the hair the exact same length on the other side.

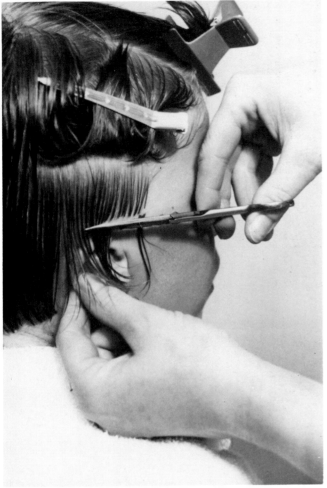

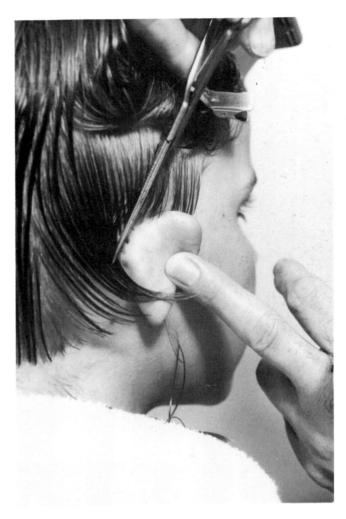

D-3 At the desired length, make a straight cut that goes to the back of the ear.

D-4 Comb the bottom corner of the nape area hair toward the ear. Folding the ear over so that it is out of the way, cut around the ear. Be sure to cut *all* the way down through the hair from the nape area that you combed forward.

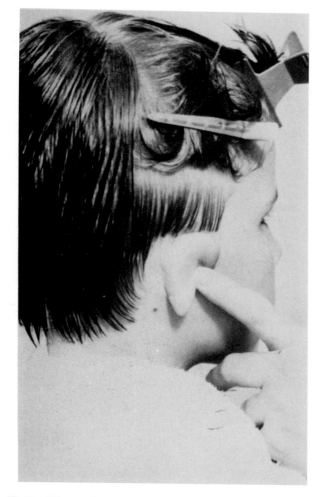

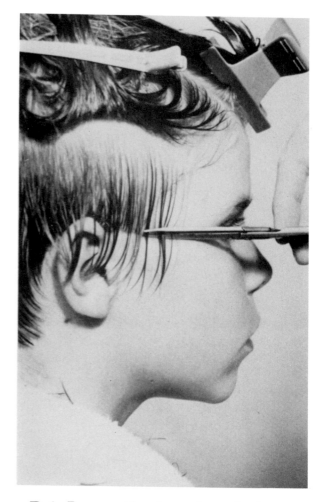

D-5 These first two cuts will serve as the guide for cutting the rest of the side.

D-6 Remove the clamp from the hair and part off another ½ inch section of hair. Cut this section following the guide hair. Continue parting off sections and cutting them the same length of the guide hair until you reach the part that runs from the front of the head to the back.

Repeat the entire procedure on the other side of the head.

CUTTING THE TOP

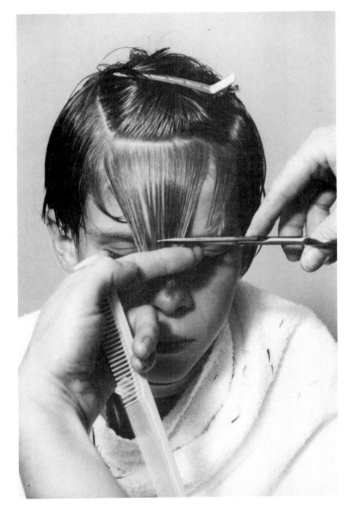

E-1   If the person whose hair you are cutting has a cowlick in the front hairline, refer to page 34.

Unclamp the hair and make a horizontal part ¾ of an inch up from the hairline that runs the entire length of the section. Using a duckbill clamp, reclamp the remaining hair to the top of the head. Comb the parted hair smoothly down. Holding it flat between your middle and index fingers, pull it down to the bridge of the nose. While holding the hair, cut it at the browline.

E-2   Usually at the sides there are some hairs that are out of line with the hair you just cut. Snip off any of these hairs that are out of line. Also snip off any hairs that are sticking below the line you cut across the forehead.

Stand behind the person and look in the mirror at the line of the front cut. This line should be straight.

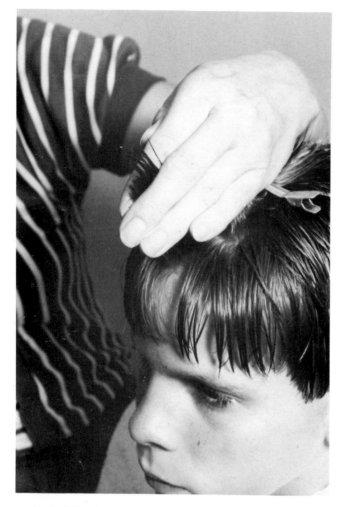

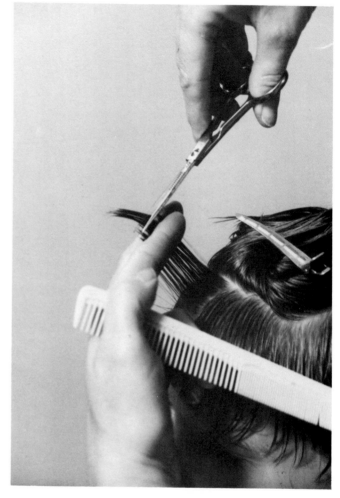

E-3 Unclamp the hair and part off another ½ inch section. Reclamp the remaining hair. In the middle of the head, pick up a vertical section of hair which includes some of the hair you previously cut.

E-4 Using the short hair in the front as your guide, cut this vertical section.

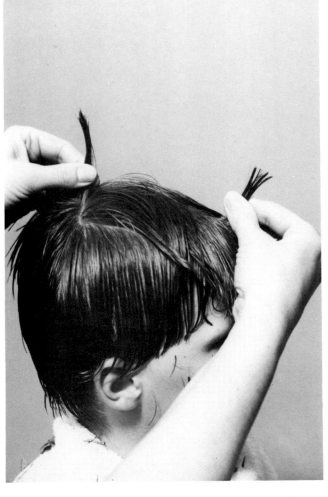

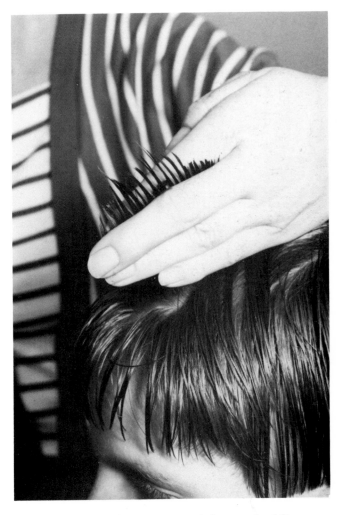

E-5 Unclamp the remaining top hair. In your right hand, pick up some of the hair from the front that you just cut and with your left hand, pick up some of the hair from the crown which was cut when you cut the back. This will show you the angle you need to cut the top in order to make it coordinate with the back.

E-6 Cut the hair in a straight vertical line from the hair you held up in the front to the hair you held up in the back. In the vertical part, use hair from the front as your guide until the section you pick up includes some of the crown hair from the back cut. Cut this section at an angle blending the two lengths together.

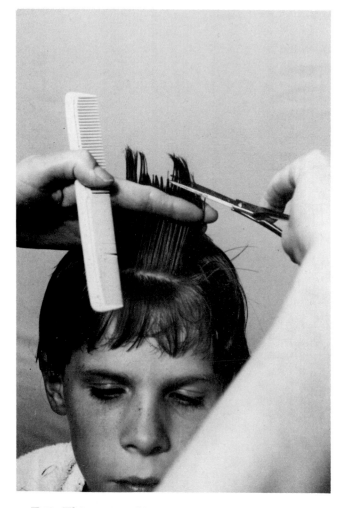

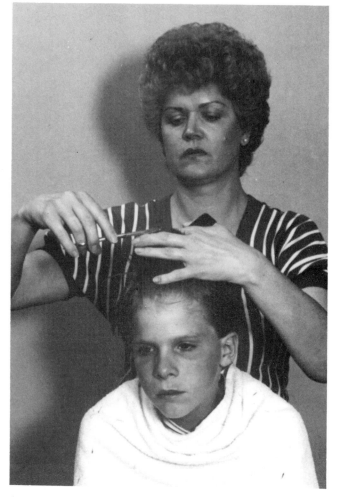

E-7 This strip of hair which runs down the center of the head will serve as the guide for cutting the rest of the top. Cut the remaining top hair, using horizontal sections, cutting the hair the same length as the middle strip.

E-8 Check the top for hairs that are longer than the desired length by picking up the hair in horizontal sections and snipping off any hairs that stick up above the rest. Be sure to check the *entire* top.

BLENDING THE TOP
AND SIDES TOGETHER

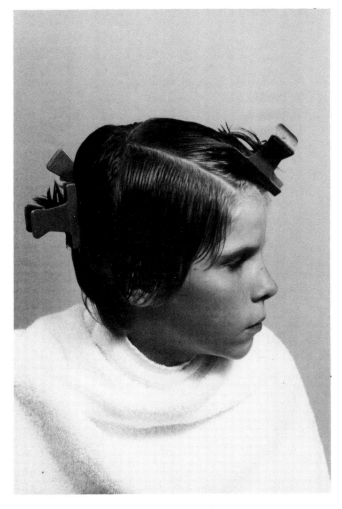

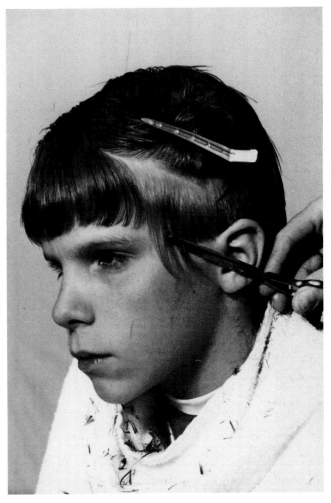

F-1 There is a strip of hair that runs just below the part which separated the top from the side that hasn't been cut yet. By cutting this strip last, you will be able to blend the top and sides together.

F-2 Make a part that angles from the top of the ear to a point an inch behind the frontal bone. Pull the hair back and clamp it in place. Comb the hair in front of the part forward and cut it, angling from the side hair to the hair in front.

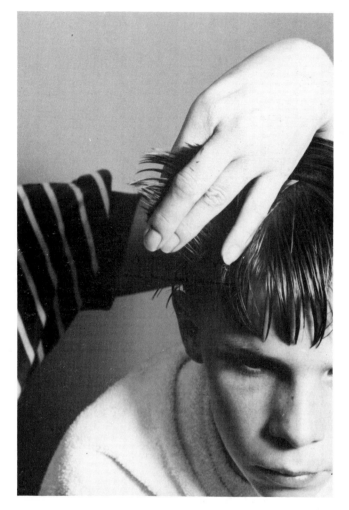

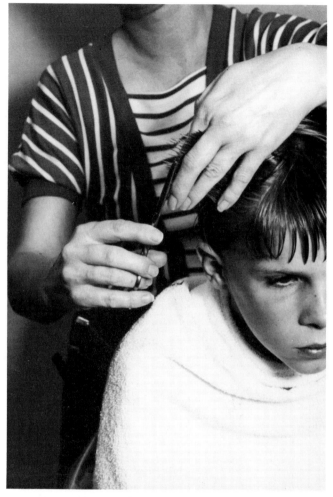

F-3 At the front of this strip, comb and part off a vertical section that includes hair that has been cut from both the top and the side. You will have short hair at both ends of the section you are holding with long uncut hair in the middle. Blend the hair from one point to the other by cutting the hair in an angle from the side hair to the top hair.

F-4 Continue cutting the hair in small sections, working your way back from the front to the back, using the hair from each previous cut as your guide.

Once you have cut the entire strip, check it the same way you checked the back and top.

Repeat the procedure on the other side.

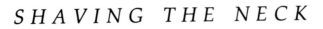

SHAVING THE NECK

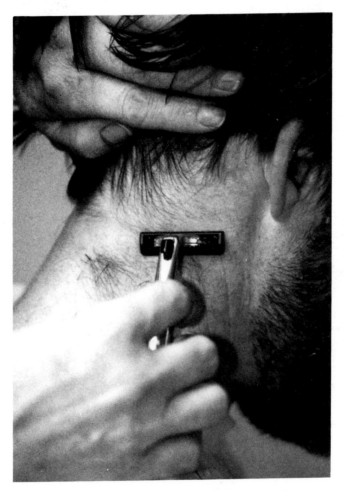

G-1 Men have hair that grows out of the back of their neck which is the equivalent of beard hair only finer. Any of this hair which is showing after the haircut needs to be shaved.

To shave this hair, clamp the nape area hair out of the way and wet or apply shaving cream to the area which is to be shaved. With a safety razor, shave the hair in a straight line.

THE BI-LEVEL

The Bi-Level is a style that many boys and young men find appealing. The Bi-Level look is achieved by cutting the sides short and leaving the back longer and layering it to achieve a fuller look. There are some particular cutting techniques that differentiate this haircut from the basic haircut.

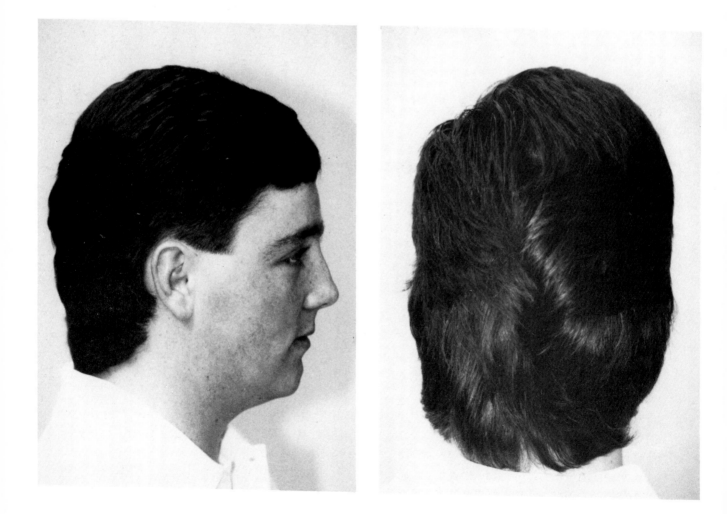

BI-LEVEL FOR STRAIGHT HAIR

CUTTING THE SIDES

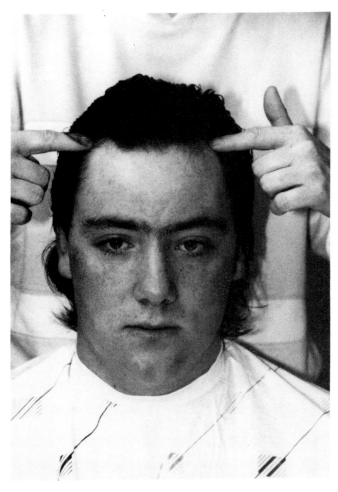

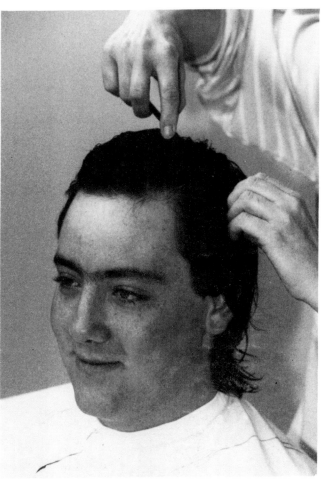

A-1 Once the hair has been washed, towel dry and comb the hair back.

It is necessary to locate the frontal bones. Feel in the hairline above the outer edges of the eyebrows until you feel the rounded edges of the frontal bones.

A-2 Starting at a frontal bone, create a part that goes straight back to the crown of the head.

Repeat this procedure on the other side.

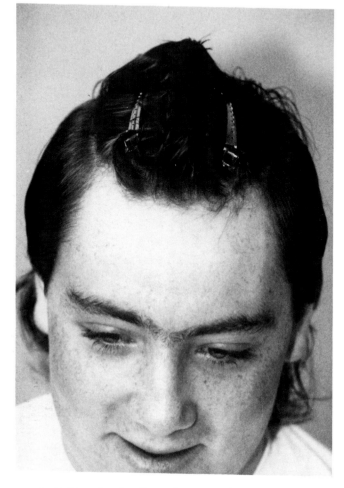

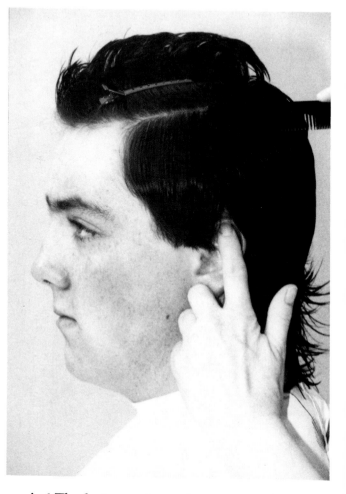

A-3 Comb the hair between these parts toward the center of the head and clamp it into place.

A-4 The hair must now be separated into front and back sections.

Place your finger on the center of the top of the ear. Create a part that runs from the frontal bone part straight down to the point you are touching on the ear.

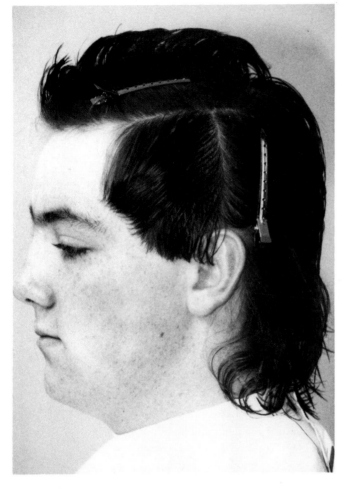

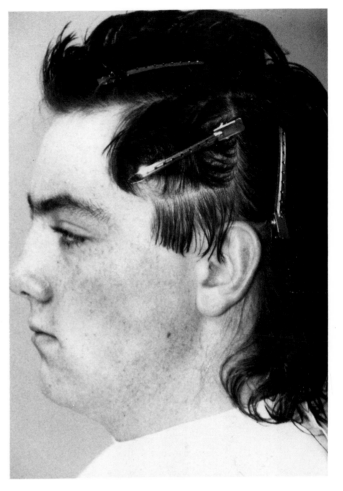

A-5 Comb the hair behind this part back. Clamp it in place.

A-6 ½ of an inch above the ear, create a horizontal part. Clamp the hair above this part into place.

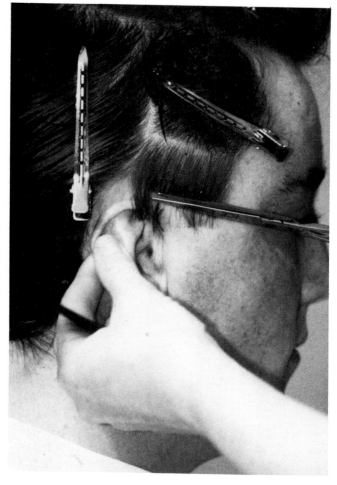 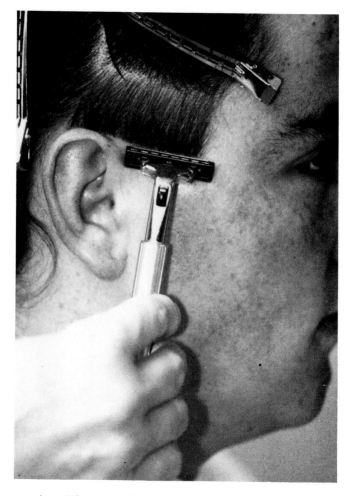

A-7 The most popular length to cut the sides for the bi-level is at a level just above the ear. However, the length of the sides depends upon personal preference.

Holding the top of the ear down so that it is out of the way, cut the side hair at the desired length. Remember to use small snips.

A-8 There will be some hair left below the line you just established with your cut. With a safety razor, shave this hair.

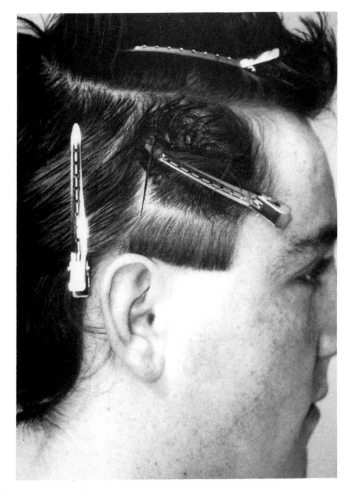

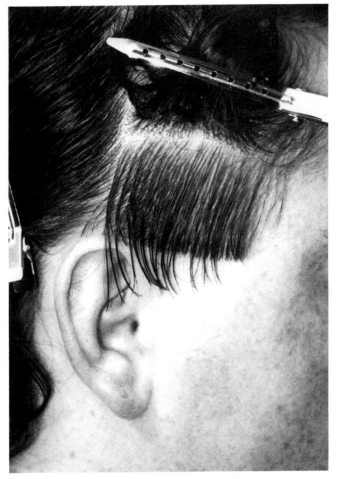

A-9 The completed cut should create a clean, straight line. This line will serve as your guide for cutting the next small section of hair.

A-10 Unclamp the side hair and create another horizontal part ½ of an inch above and parallel with the last part. Clamp the hair above this part back into place.

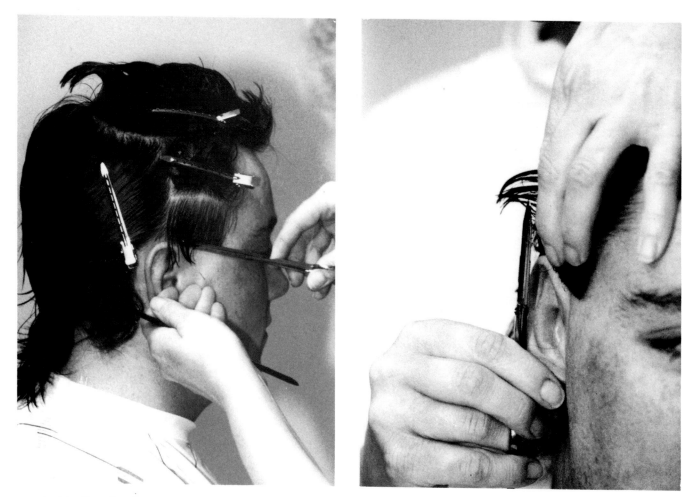

A-11 Comb the unclamped hair down and cut it by placing the scissors at a level just below the guide hair.

Part off one more ½ inch horizontal section and cut it the same way you cut the last section.

A-12 Starting at the front of the side hair, pick up a ½ inch vertical section of hair and place it between your second and third fingers. This section should run from the bottom of the side straight up to the horizontal part.

Hold this hair snug and straight out from the head. Cut it, using small snips and moving straight up from the shortest hair which is at the bottom. Cutting the hair this way will layer it.

Moving toward the back of the head, pick up another ½ inch vertical section of hair. Be sure to include some of the hair you just cut. Cut this hair using the previously cut hair as your guide.

Continue cutting the hair in vertical sections until you reach the part that divides the front from the back. Remember to always use the hair that you just previously cut as a guide for cutting each new section.

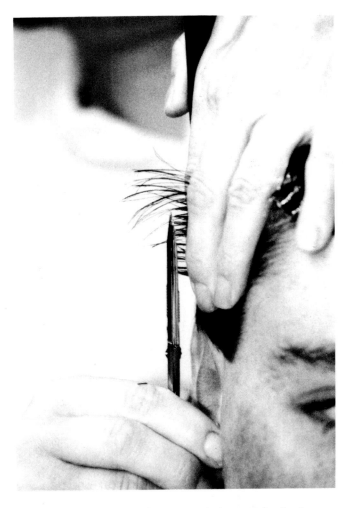

A-13 Unclamp the remaining side hair and comb it down. Begin at the front of the side and cut this hair in vertical sections using the same technique that you used to cut the lower portion of the side.

Repeat this process on the other side beginning with step A-4.

C U T T I N G   T H E   B A C K

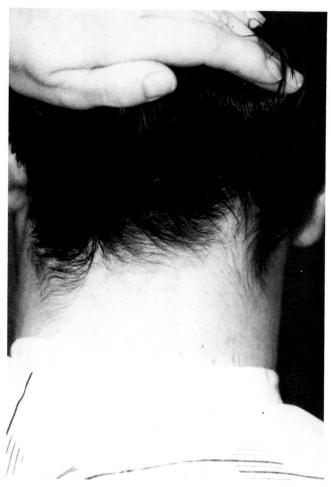

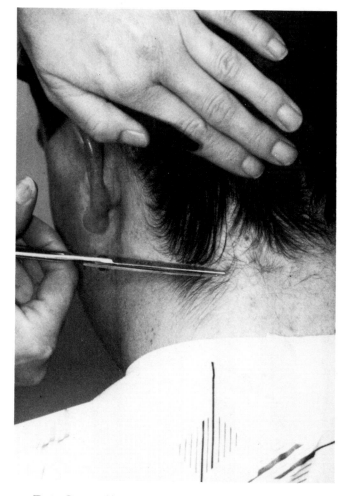

B-1 Lift the hair up off the back of the neck so that you can clearly see the growth line of the hair on the neck. On many men this line is very uneven and includes a cowlick or two.

B-2 Cut off any hair that is out of line with the back growth line. To do this, take the scissors and cut across the back, rounding the sides up slightly.

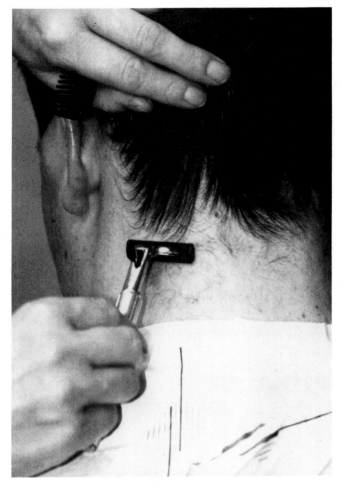

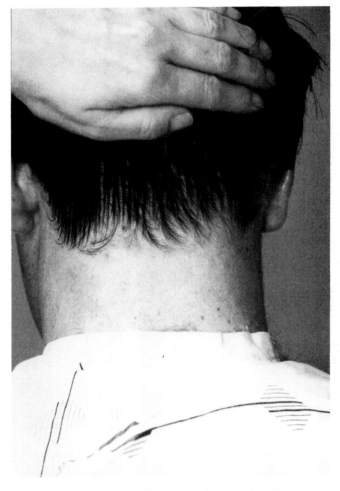

B-3 After you have established a nice even line with your scissors, use a safety razor to shave off any hair that lies below this line.

B-4 The growth line on the back of the neck should now be clean and even and slightly rounded at the corners.

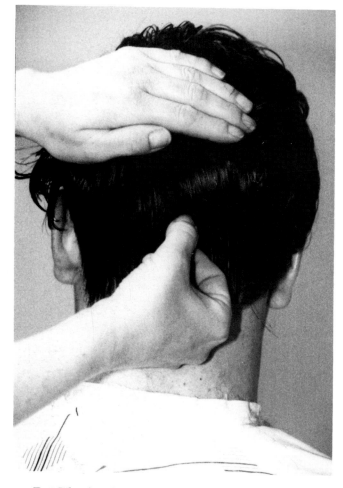

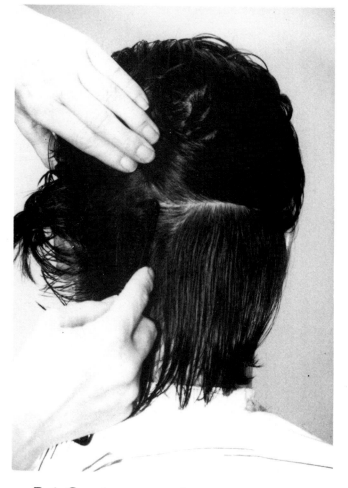

B-5 The back must now be separated into top and bottom sections. To do this, you must locate the occipital bone.

The occipital bone forms the base of the skull. To locate it, feel the back of the head until you find where the skull curves in. The large bone you feel at this point is the occipital bone.

B-6 Create a part that runs straight across the back, just below the occipital bone.

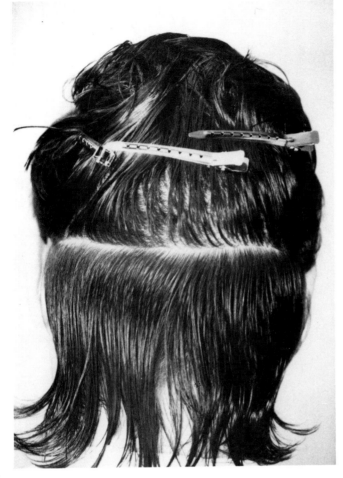

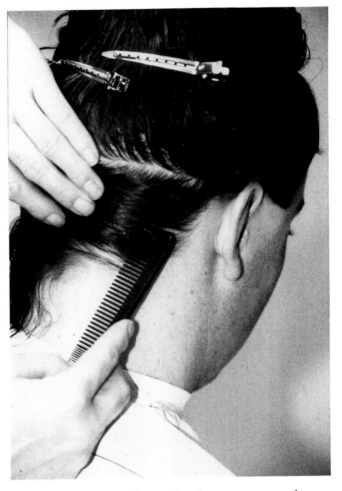

B-7 Clamp the hair above this part using duckbill clamps. The back of the head is now divided into top and bottom sections. The area below the part is called the nape area.

B-8 1 inch up from the bottom growth line, create a horizontal part that runs straight across the nape area.

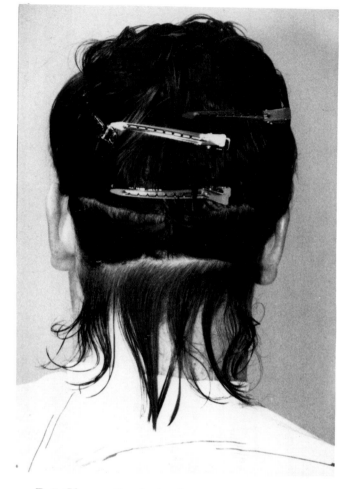

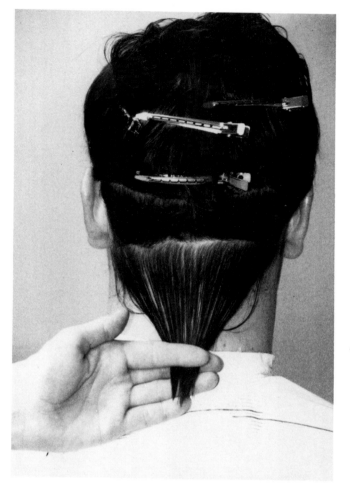

B-9 Clamp the hair above this part with a duckbill clamp.

B-10 Gather the unclamped hair into a "V" and place the end of the "V" in the middle of the neck. Holding the hair snug and straight down, cut it at the desired length.

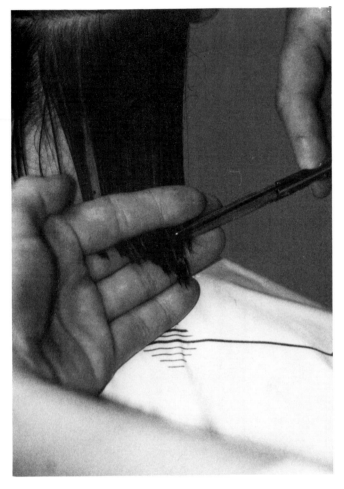

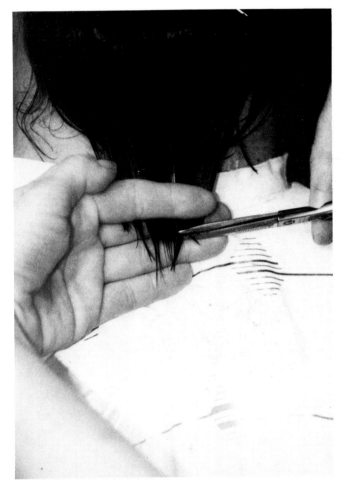

B-11 Because this hair was cut while pulling it to the center, some of the hair on the sides of the back were not cut. Place the hair from one side between your second and third fingers. Place your third finger against the neck. Cut this hair, rounding the corner and following the line established by the hair that has already been cut.

B-12 Unclamp the nape area hair and create a part ½ of an inch above the last part. Re-clamp the hair above the new part.

Gather all the unclamped hair into a "V." Hold this hair snug and cut it using the previously cut hair as your guide.

Round the hair on the sides of this section following the guide.

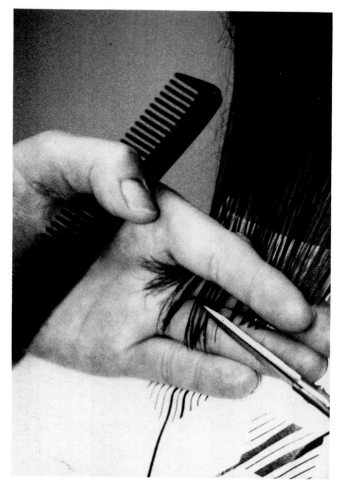

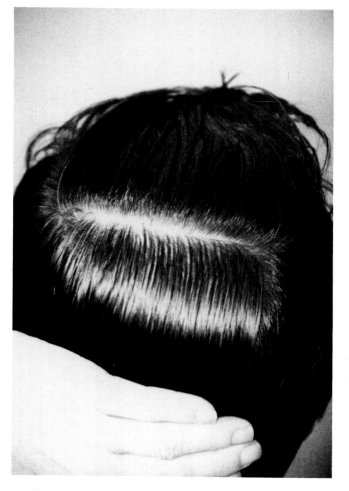

B-13 Unclamp the remaining nape area hair and comb it down. Beginning on one side of this hair, pick up a finger length of hair and hold it between your second and third fingers. With your third finger resting on the neck, pull the hair down snug. Cut this hair using the previously cut hair as your guide. Continue cutting finger lengths of hair, working from one side to the other.

B-14 Unclamp the top half of the back and comb it smoothly down. Create a part that runs straight across the crown of the head.

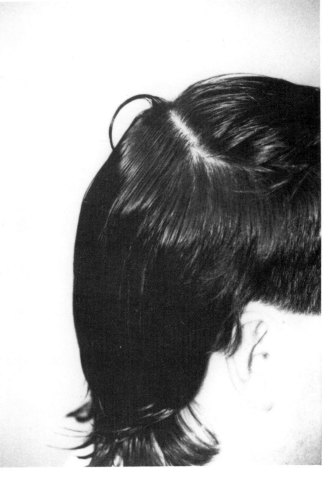

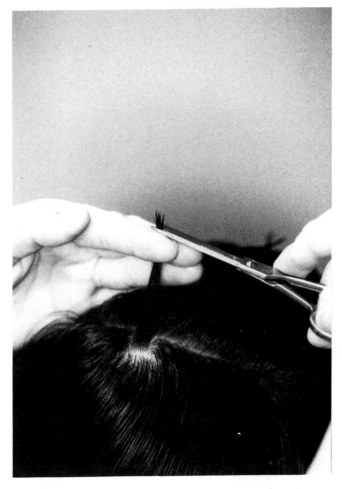

B-15 In the center of the crown of the head, pick up a ¼ inch section of hair. Run this hair between your fingers until it sticks together. Holding this hair straight up from the head, let go of it and it will fall back to the head, forming an arch.

B-16 Take hold of this hair and cut it at the exact point where it touches the head. This technique ensures that the crown hair is cut the proper length for the individual.

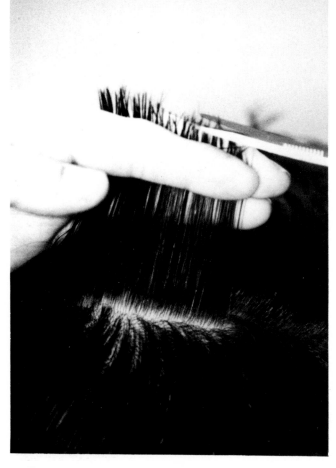

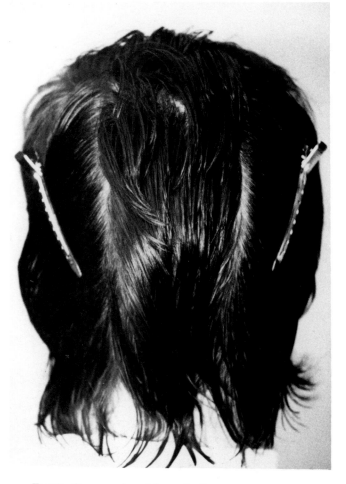

B-17 Pick up a finger length of hair that includes the ¼ inch section of hair that you just cut. Cut this section of hair using the short, previously cut hair as a guide.

B-18 On each side of the section you just cut, create a vertical part that runs straight down the back of the head. The strip of hair that lies between these two parts will be cut next. Clamp the hair on each side of this strip forward and out of the way.

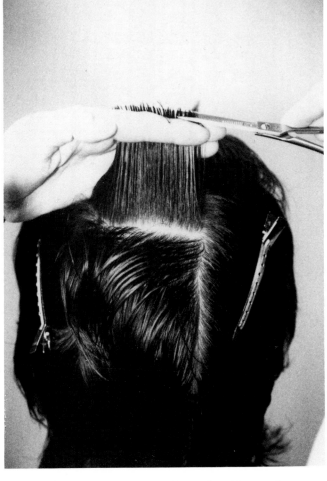

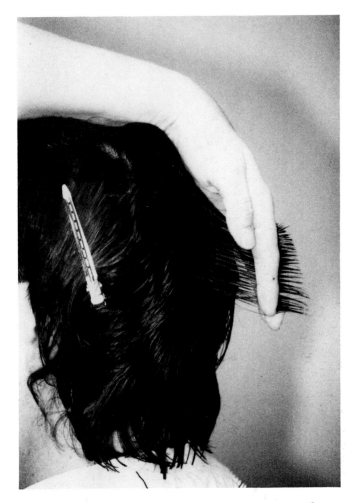

B-19 Pick up a finger length of hair that runs parallel with the crown and includes some of the hair that you have already cut. Holding this hair straight up from the head, cut it, using the previously cut hair as your guide.

Working your way down the back, continue parting off and cutting horizontal sections, always including some of the hair from the previously cut section to use as your guide.

As you work your way down, eventually the hair you lift up will already be shorter than your guide. When this happens, move on to the next step.

B-20 At the place where you stopped cutting the hair in horizontal sections, pick up a vertical section of hair, in the middle of the center strip. Hold this hair straight out from the head, then lower it slightly. This will place the hair on a slight angle.

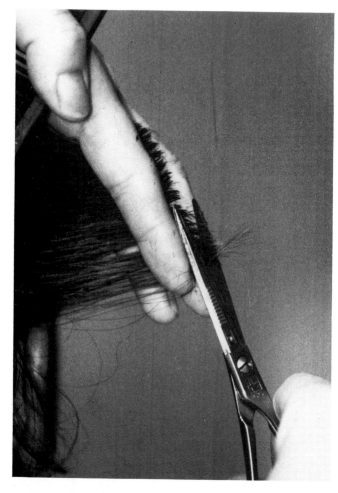

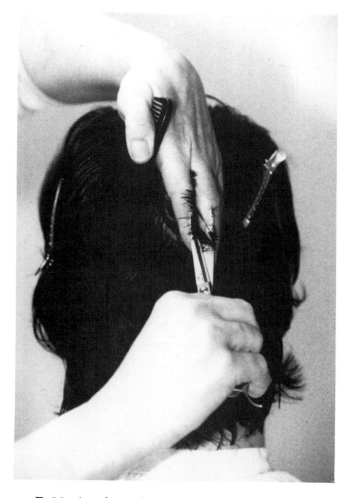

B-21 Cut this hair on an angle from the long hair at the bottom of the section to the short hair at the top.

Moving down the back in a straight line, continue picking up vertical sections of hair and cutting them the same way as the first section. Keep doing this until you reach the bottom.

B-22 At the place where you started cutting the hair in vertical sections, move slightly to one side of the vertical section you just cut and begin picking up and cutting vertical sections again. Include some hair from the previously cut strip to serve as your guide.

Continue cutting the back in small vertical strips until the entire bottom has been cut.

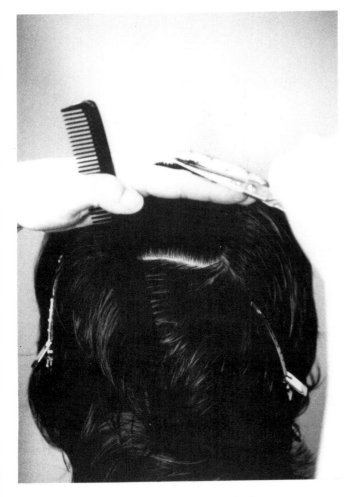

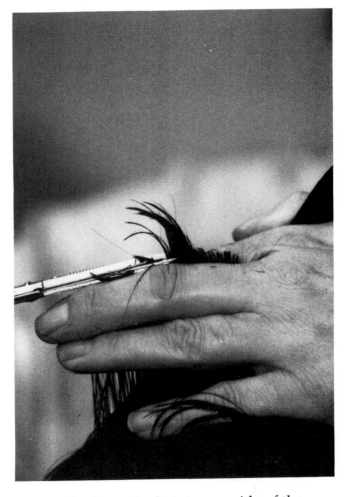

B-23 Go back to the top of the center strip and check the hair to make sure that it is even. To do this, begin at the top and pick up horizontal sections of hair, snipping off any hairs that stick up above the rest.

B-24 Unclamp the hair to one side of the center strip and comb it down. Pick up a ½ inch wide horizontal section of this hair that runs from the side part, over to and including some of the hair from the center strip that you have already cut. Use the previously cut hair as your guide to cut this hair. The hair that you just cut will serve as your guide for cutting the rest of this third of the back.

Cut the rest of this section using the same technique you used to cut the center strip. See steps B-19 through B-21.

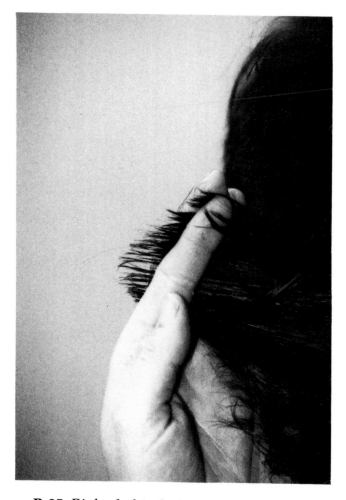

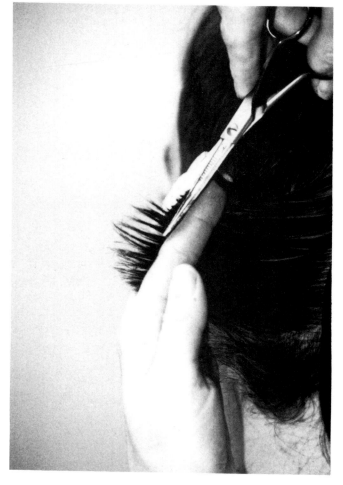

B-25 Right behind the ear, pick up a vertical section of hair and place it between your second and third fingers. Hold this hair straight out from the head, then pull it around to the side. Holding the hair this way will allow you to see a small section of hair that sticks out further than the rest.

B-26 Cut off this hair following the line of the hair between your fingers that has already been cut.

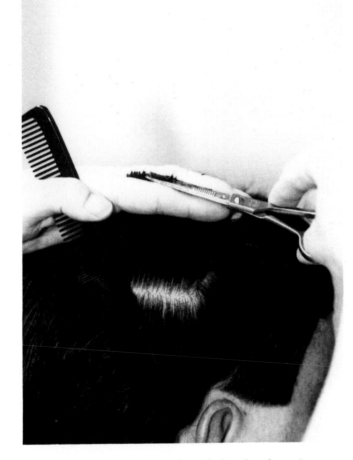

B-27 Check this side of the back using the same technique you used on the center strip.

Repeat this entire procedure on the hair that lies on the other side of the center strip beginning at B-24. The back is now complete.

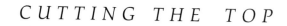

CUTTING THE TOP

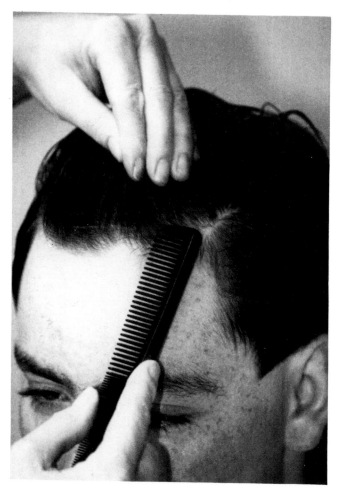

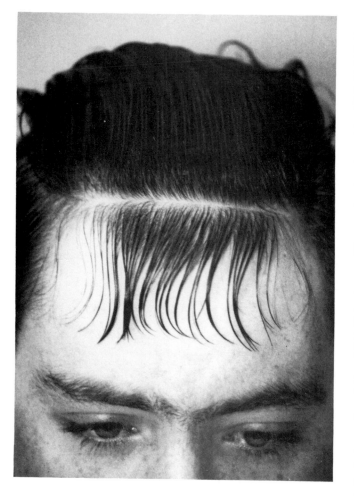

C-1 Unclamp the top hair. ½ of an inch behind the hairline, create a part that runs straight across the front of the head.

C-2 Comb the hair behind the part back. Comb the hair in front of the part straight down. The completed part should be straight and distinct.

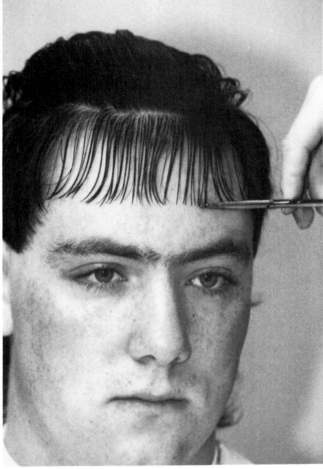

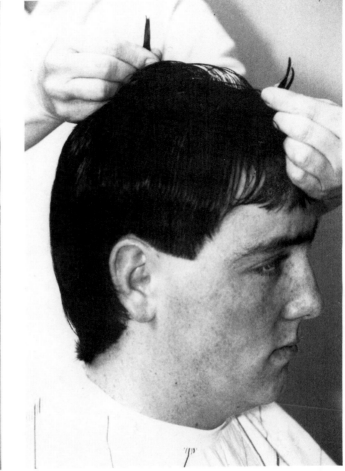

C-3 If the front hair is longer than eye-brow level, refer to steps E-1 and E-2 of the basic haircut. If the front hair is shorter than the eyebrow level, cut the hair at the desired length, taking small snips and cutting straight across the front.

½ of an inch behind the first part, create another horizontal part. Comb the hair down. You should be able to see the previously cut hair underneath to use as your guide. Place your scissors just below the guide hair and cut.

C-4 In the middle of the front of the head pick up a small piece of the hair you just cut. At the crown of the head, straight back from the front hair you are holding up, pick up a small piece of the crown hair that you cut when you were cutting the back. These two pieces show the angle that you need to cut the center strip which will serve as your guide for cutting the top.

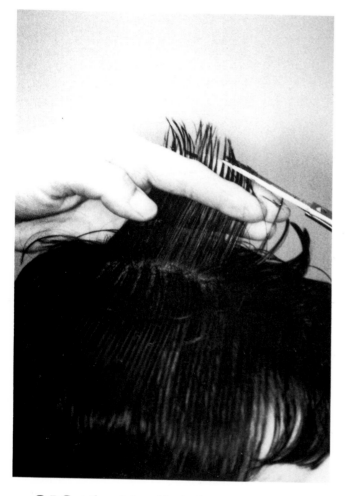

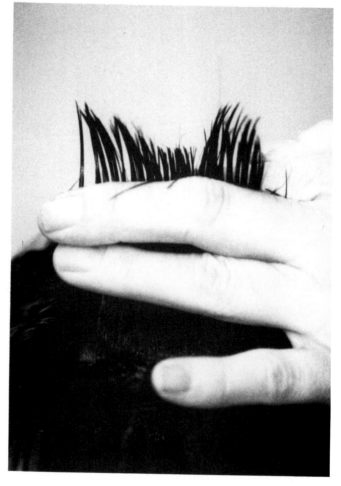

C-5 Cut the strip of hair that lies between these two points by picking up narrow vertical sections and cutting them following the angle established by the two small pieces of hair.

C-6 At the front of the strip you just cut, pick up a horizontal section of hair. In the middle of this section you will be able to see the hair of the strip you just cut. Cut this section using the previously cut hair as your guide.

Continue parting off ½ inch horizontal sections and cutting them the same length as the center strip until you reach the crown.

Check the top by picking up horizontal sections and snipping off any hairs that were missed the first time.

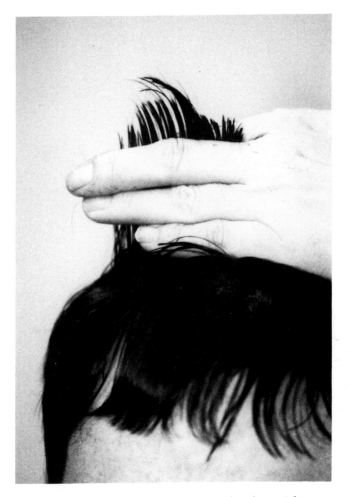

C-7 To blend the top with the side, pick up a finger length of hair just behind the part that sectioned off the front hair. This section should include hair from the top and hair from the side section that you cut earlier.

Holding this hair up straight from the head, cut it on an angle going from the length of the side hair to the length of the top hair.

Continue cutting finger lengths of hair, moving back until you reach the crown.

Repeat this step on the other side.

The haircut is now complete.

BI-LEVEL FOR CURLY HAIR

The Bi-Level style looks very good with curly hair. Whether the curl is natural or achieved through a permanent, the technique for cutting the back is somewhat different than that of cutting the back on straight hair.

Instructions for perming the hair for the Bi-Level are given later in this chapter.

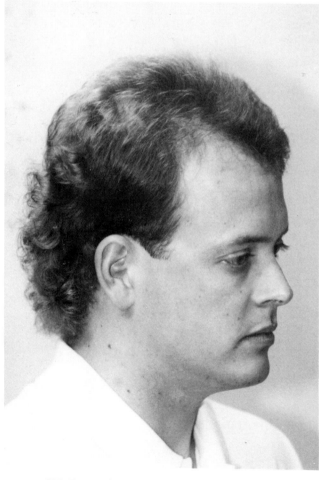

Bi-Level on Permed Hair

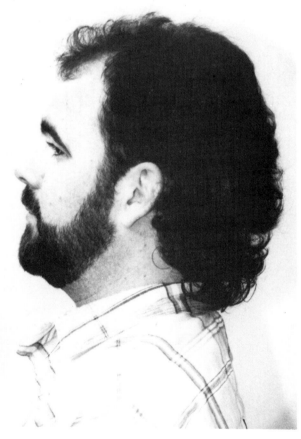

Bi-Level on Naturally Curly Hair

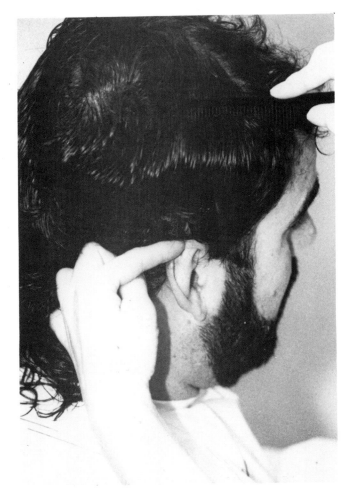

A-1 The hair must be separated into front and back sections. To do this, place your finger at the top of the ear. Create a part that runs from the point you are touching on the ear, straight up the side of the head, over the top of the head and straight down to the same point on the other ear.

A-2 Clamp the hair in front of this part with a duckbill clamp.

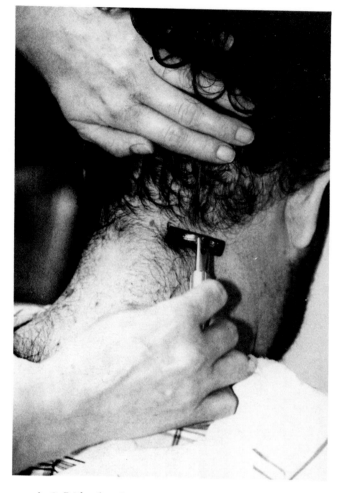

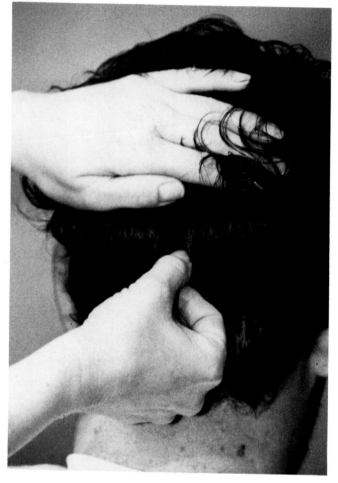

A-3 Lift the hair up off the back of the neck so you can clearly see the growth line of the hair on the neck. With a safety razor, clean up the back of the neck, removing any hair below the growth line.

A-4 The back must be separated into top and bottom sections. To do this, you must locate the occipital bone.

The occipital bone forms the base of the skull. To locate it, feel the back of the head until you find the point where the skull curves in. The large bone you feel at this point is the occipital bone.

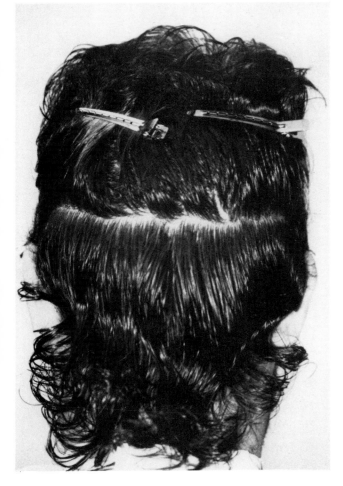

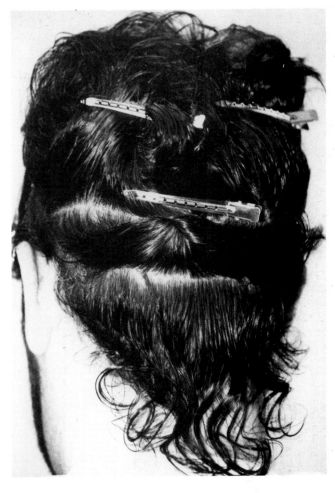

A-5 Create a part that runs straight across the back of the head just below the occipital bone. Clamp the hair above the part in place with duckbill clamps.

The back of the head is now divided into top and bottom sections. The area below the part is called the nape area.

A-6 1 inch up from the bottom growth line of the hair, create a horizontal part that runs straight across the nape area. Twist and clamp the hair above this part with a duckbill clamp.

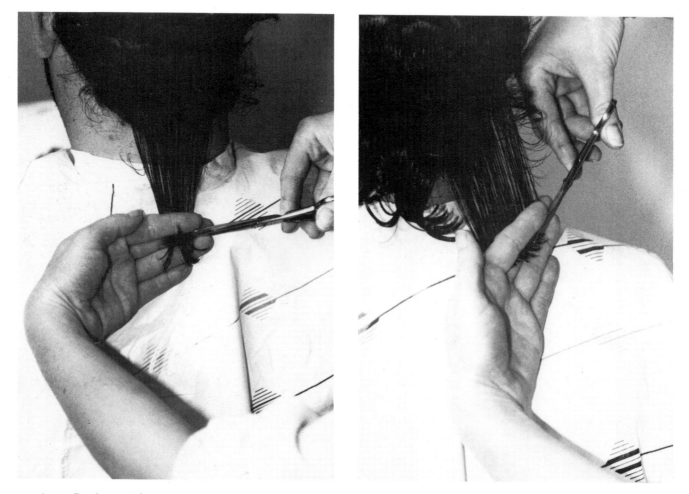

A-7 Gather the unclamped nape area hair into a "V" and place the end of the "V" on the spine. Holding this hair straight down, cut it. Because curly hair will pull up when it dries, be sure to cut the hair at a length that is a little longer than the desired length.

A-8 Because this hair was cut while pulling it to the center, some of the hair on the sides of the back were not cut. Place the hair from one side between your second and third fingers. Place your third finger against the neck. Cut this hair, rounding the corner and following the line established by the hair that has already been cut.

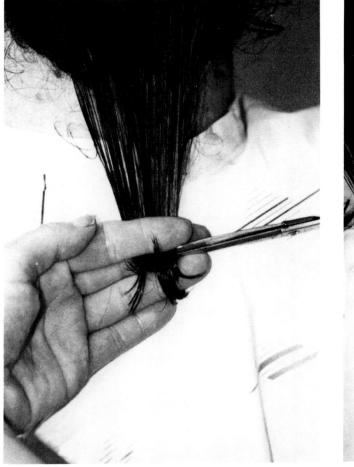

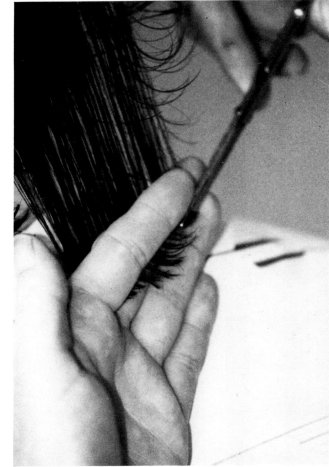

A-9 Unclamp the nape area hair and create a part ½ of an inch above the last part. Re-clamp the hair above the new part.

Gather all the unclamped hair into a "V." Hold this hair snug and cut it, using the previously cut hair as your guide.

Round the hair on the sides of this section following the guide.

A-10 Unclamp the remaining nape area hair and comb it down. Beginning on one side of this hair, pick up a finger length of hair and hold it between your second and third fingers. With your third finger resting on the neck, pull the hair down snug. Cut this hair using the previously cut hair as your guide. Continue cutting finger lengths of hair, working from one side to the other.

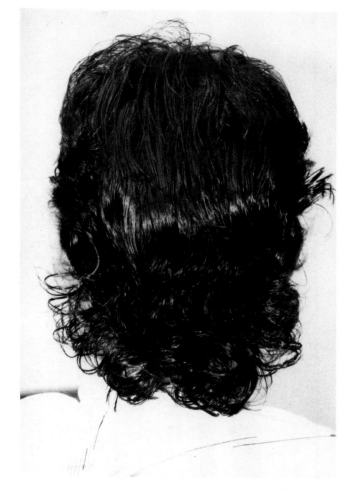

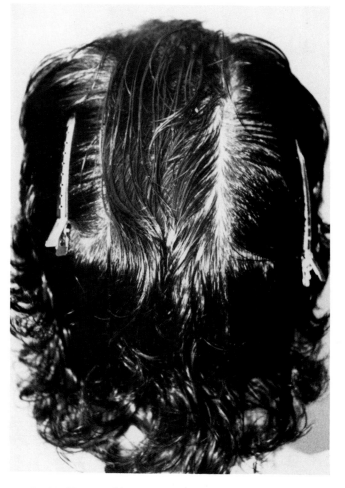

A-11 Unclamp the top half of the back and comb the hair down smoothly.

A-12 Part off a 2½ inch strip running from the crown all the way down the back of the head. Clamp the hair on both sides of this strip forward.

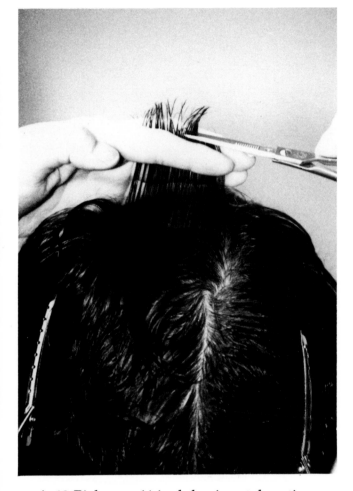

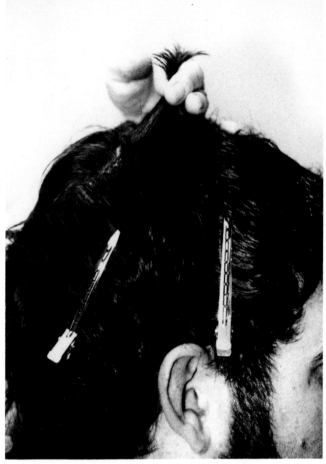

A-13 Pick up a ½ inch horizontal section at the top of the center strip. Holding the hair snug and straight up, cut it at a length 2 inches above the head. When released, the cut hair should stand up.

A-14 Pull up another ½ inch section of hair. Include in this section some of the hair from the section you just cut. Hold this hair straight up from the head then pull it slightly forward. Cut this hair using the previously cut hair as your guide.

Working your way down the back, continue parting off and cutting horizontal ½ inch sections. Always hold the hair straight up and a little forward from the top of the head. Eventually, the hair you hold up will already be shorter than the guide. When this happens, move on to the next step.

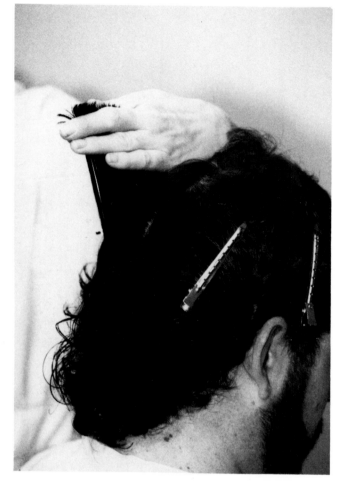

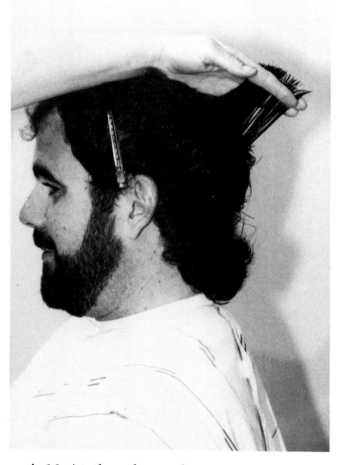

A-15 At the place where you stopped cutting the hair in horizontal sections, pick up a vertical section of hair in the middle of the center strip. Hold this hair snug and straight out from the head, then raise it slightly.

Cut this hair on an angle from the long hair at the bottom of the section to the short hair at the top.

Moving down the back in a straight line, continue picking up vertical sections of hair and cutting them the same way as the first section. Keep doing this until you reach the bottom.

A-16 At the place where you started cutting the hair in vertical sections, move slightly to one side of the vertical section you just cut and begin picking up and cutting vertical sections again. Include some hair from the previously cut strip to serve as your guide.

Continue cutting the back in small vertical strips until the entire bottom of the center strip has been cut.

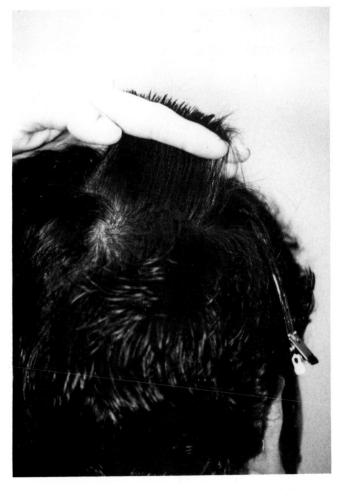

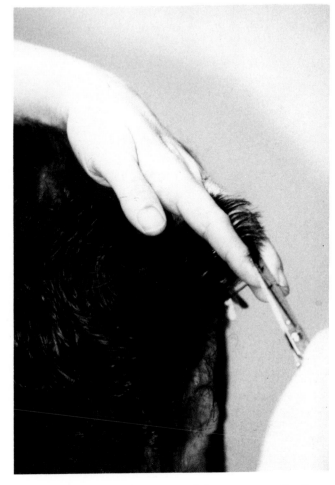

A-17 Unclamp the hair to one side of the center strip and comb it down. Pick up a ½ inch wide horizontal section of this hair that runs from the side part, over to and including some of the hair from the center strip that you have already cut. Use the previously cut hair as your guide to cut this hair. The hair that you just cut will serve as your guide for cutting the rest of this third of the back.

Cut the rest of this section using the same technique you used to cut the center strip. See Steps A-14 through A-16.

A-18 Behind the ear, pick up a vertical section of hair and place it between your second and third fingers. Hold this hair straight out from the head, then pull it around to the side. Holding the hair this way will allow you to see a small section of hair that sticks out further than the rest. Cut off this hair following the line established by the hair which you are holding that has already been cut.

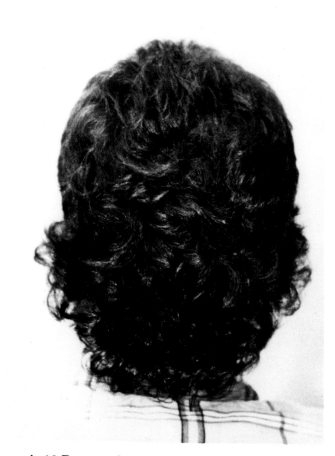

A-19 Repeat this entire procedure on the hair that lies on the other side of the center strip, beginning at A-17.

The back is now complete. The sides and top can be cut following the instructions found in the Bi-Level for straight hair. See pages 37-43, 58-61.

PERMING THE HAIR FOR THE BI-LEVEL

Rolling a perm is not difficult if you take your time and do it in an organized fashion. For the Bi-Level, the back is the only hair that you perm. The top and sides are cut short and do not require perming. It is always best to perm the hair first and then cut it.

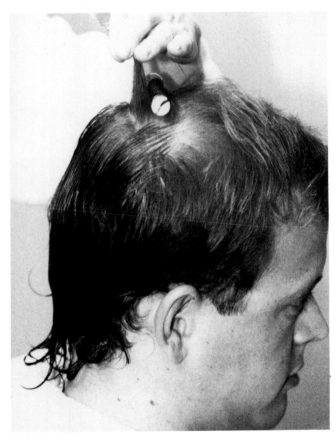

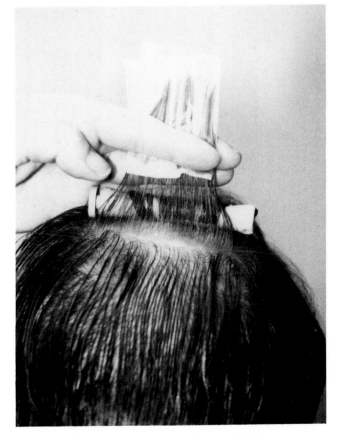

A-1 Beginning in the center of the back at the crown, pick up a horizontal section of hair that is approximately the length of a perm rod.

A-2 While holding this hair, fold a tissue over the hair. Slide the tissue to the end of the hair. None of the hair should stick out past the end of the tissue. Place the rod at the end of the tissue and begin wrapping. It is essential that you roll the rod with the same amount of pressure on both sides of the rod.

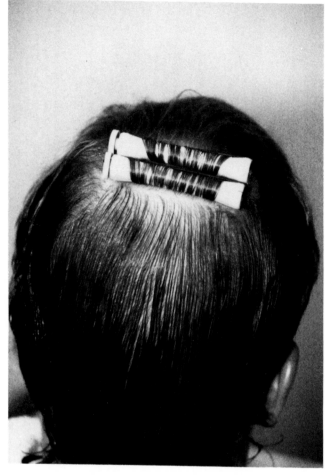

A-3 Keep the hair wet throughout the rolling process by spraying it with water. Do not attempt to roll the hair if it is not wet.

A-4 Continue rolling sections of hair so that the rods form a straight line down the back of the head.

When the center strip is complete, roll the hair that lies on both sides of the center. The back is now complete and ready for the solution to be applied.

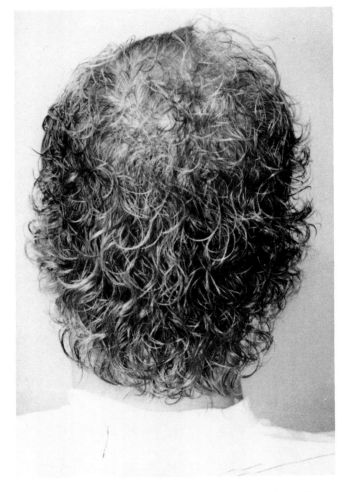

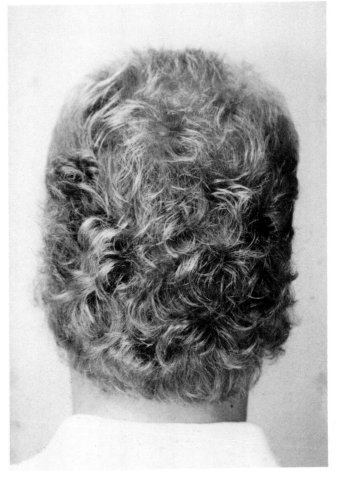

A-5 After the hair has been permed and is still wet, it is ready to be cut.

A-6 The hair after it has been permed and cut.

TROUBLE AREAS

Obviously, everyone's hair grows differently. Sometimes the way a person's hair grows presents a problem for cutting the hair. This chapter identifies the most common of these growth patterns and explains how to cut them to obtain the best results.

COWLICK IN THE FRONT HAIRLINE

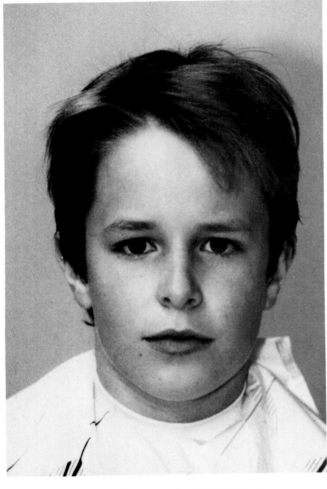

A-1 A cowlick is a tuft of hair that grows contrary to the growth pattern of the rest of the hair. Because of this, the hair will not lie down smoothly. Therefore, you must cut the front differently if there is a cowlick in the hairline.

A-2 ½ inch back from the front hairline, create a horizontal part. Comb this hair smoothly down, clamp the hair behind the part into place.

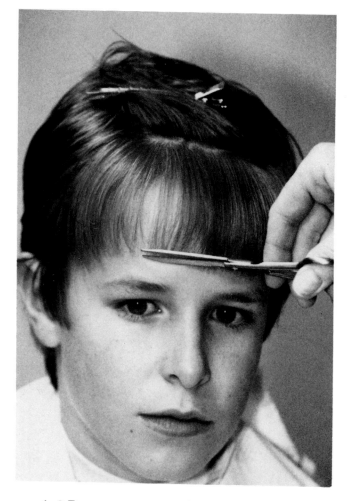 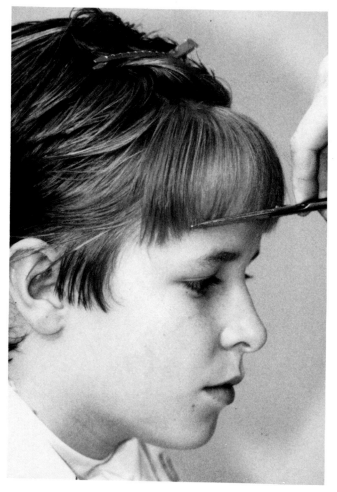

A-3 Because you need to see the cowlick clearly, make sure the hair is only slightly damp when you cut it.

Never force the cowlick down so that it conforms with the other hair while you cut it. This is a sure way to get an uneven cut.

Cut the cowlick at the desired length. This will serve as your guide for cutting the rest of the front.

A-4 From the cowlick, work to the side, cutting the hair with small snips, straight across.

As you cut around to the side, curve the line you are cutting slightly down.

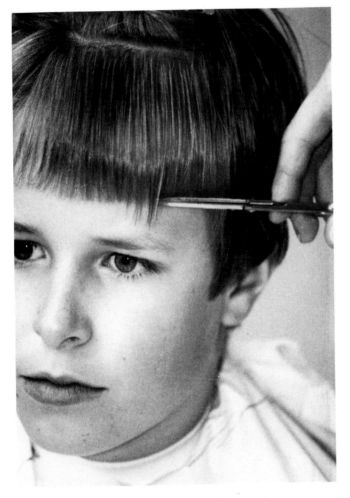

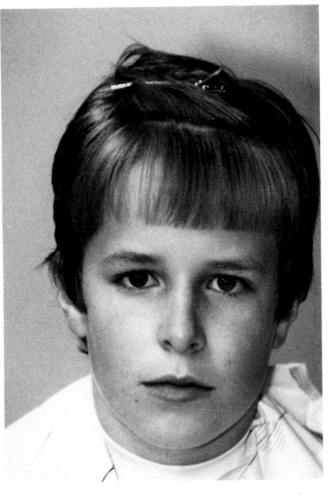

A-5 Starting from the other side, cut around to the cowlick. Be sure to follow the line that you have already established.

A-6 The finished cut should be even and straight.

Unclamp the hair and part off another ½ inch section. Comb this hair straight down. Clamp the hair behind this part back into place.

Cut this hair by placing the scissors slightly below the previously cut hair and snip along the line established by the previously cut hair.

You have now successfully dealt with the cowlick. Finish cutting the hair by following the instructions from the desired haircut.

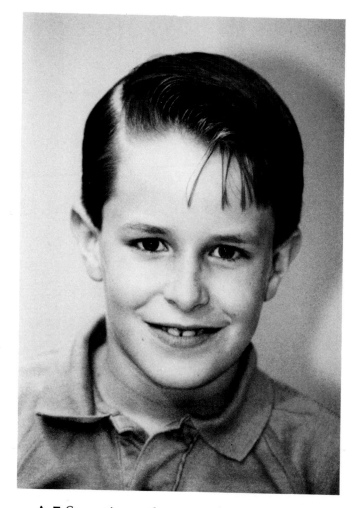

A-7 Sometimes the growth pattern of a cowlick can be incorporated in the styling of the hair.

CUTTING A DOUBLE CROWN

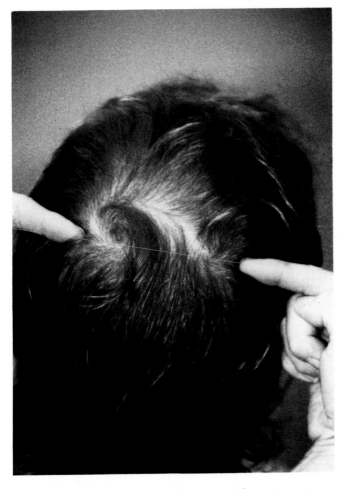

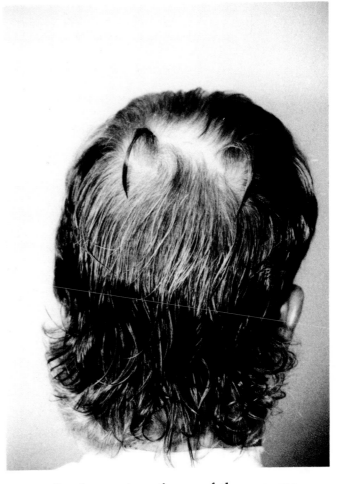

A-1 The crown is the central point at which the hair grows out of the head. If a person has a double crown, like this model, you must use a different technique than when you cut hair with a single crown.

A-2 In the center of one of the crowns, pick up a ¼ inch section of hair. Run this hair between your fingers until it sticks together. Holding this hair straight up from the head, let go of it and it will fall back to the head, forming an arch.

Repeat this procedure on the other crown. There should now be two arches falling back to the head.

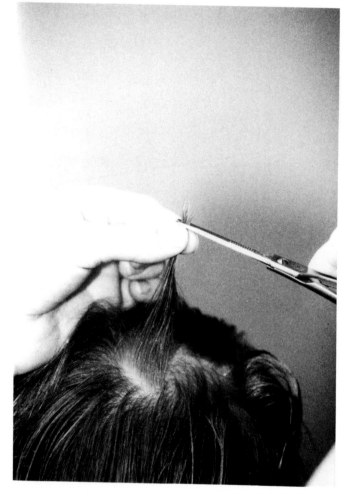

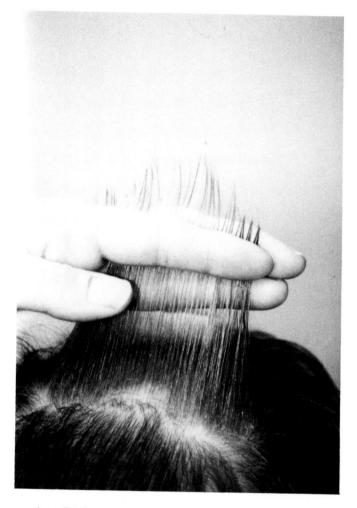

A-3 Take hold of one of these arches and cut it at the exact point where it touched the head.

Repeat this procedure on the hair of the other arch.

A-4 Pick up a ½ inch horizontal section that runs from crown to crown.
On each side of this section you should be able to see the cut hair from the two arches.

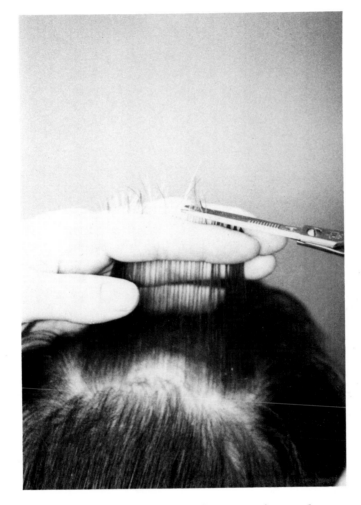

A-5 Cut, straight and even, from the short hair on one side to the short hair on the other side.

This section will serve as your guide for cutting the rest of the back. You can now cut the rest of the back following the instructions from the desired haircut.

RECEDING AND THINNING HAIR

Thinning or receding hair needs to be cut differently than a full head of hair. The recession and thinning areas need to be compensated for in order to achieve the best look for the individual.

A common mistake men often make is letting their hair grow long. They think that the length will make up for the fullness they lack. This is a mistake because it actually makes the hair look thinner than it is.

CUTTING THE SIDES

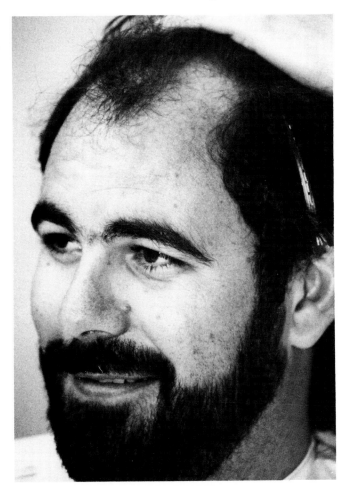

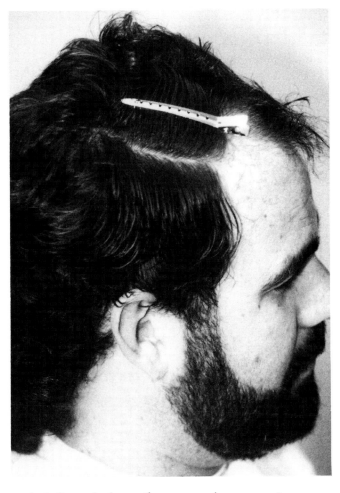

A-1 This model has a definite recession and is thinning on top.

A-2 Just below the recession, create a part that goes straight to a point that is even with the crown of the head. Clamp the hair above the part with a duckbill clamp.

Repeat this procedure on the other side.

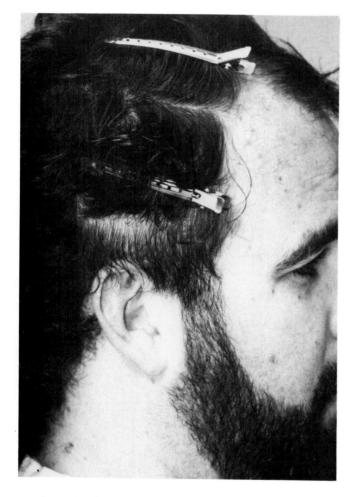

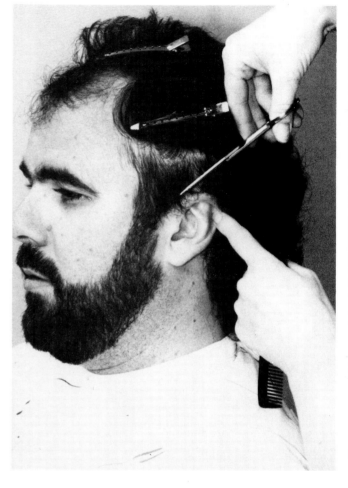

A-3 ½ of an inch above the ear, create a horizontal part. Clamp the hair above the part with a duckbill clamp.

A-4 Holding the top of the ear out of the way, cut the side hair at the desired length. Remember that short hair is better for thinning hair.

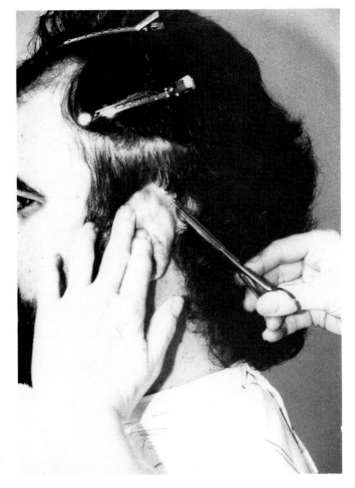

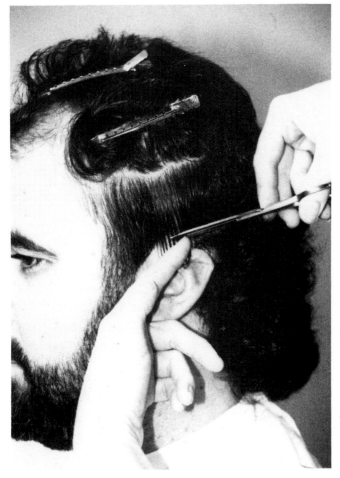

A-5 Fold the ear over so that you can cut the hair behind the ear the desired length.

A-6 Unclamp the side hair and create another horizontal part ½ of an inch above and parallel with the last part. Clamp the hair above this part back into place.

Cut this hair by placing the scissors slightly below the previously cut hair and cut, following the line you established when you made the first cut.

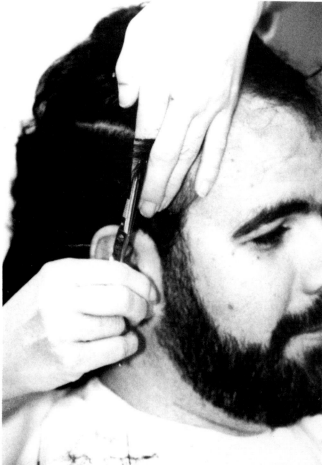

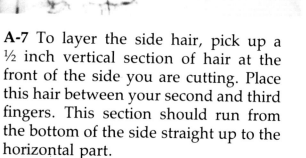

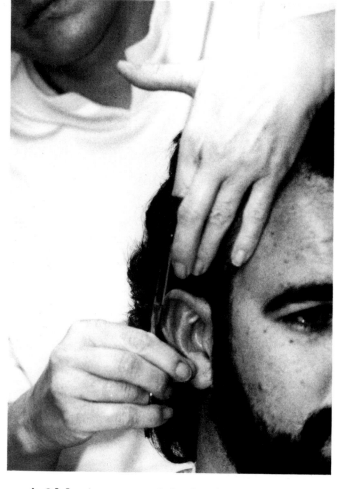

A-7 To layer the side hair, pick up a ½ inch vertical section of hair at the front of the side you are cutting. Place this hair between your second and third fingers. This section should run from the bottom of the side straight up to the horizontal part.

Holding this hair straight out from the head, cut it, using small snips, moving straight up from the shortest hair at the bottom.

A-8 Moving toward the back of the head, pick up another ½ inch vertical section, making sure to include some of the hair you just cut. Cut this hair, using the previously cut hair as your guide for the length.

Continue cutting the hair in vertical sections until you reach the back. Remember to always use the hair that you just previously cut as the guide for cutting each new section.

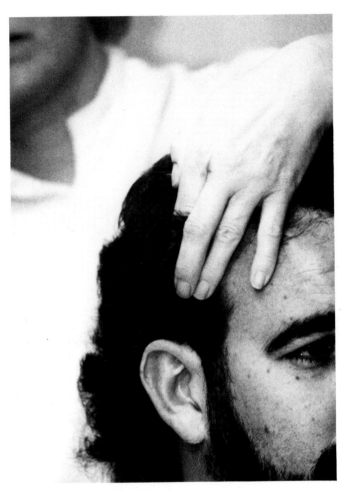

A-9 Unclamp the remaining side hair and comb it down. Beginning at the front, cut this hair in vertical sections, using the same technique you used to cut the lower portion of the side.

Repeat this process on the other side, beginning with step A-2.

CUTTING THE TOP

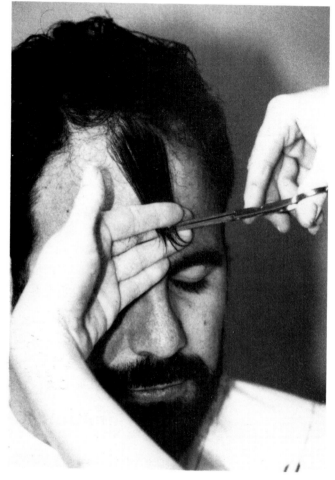

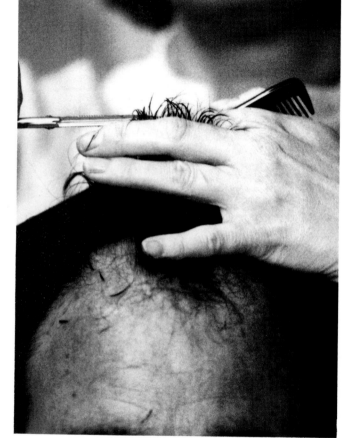

B-1 Unclamp the hair on top of the head. ½ of an inch behind the front hairline create a horizontal part. This part should be parallel with the hairline and as straight as possible.

Pull the hair into a "V" and hold it between your second and third fingers. Pull this hair down snug and cut it at a level that is slightly longer than the desired length.

B-2 Part off another horizontal ½ inch wide strip of hair that includes some of the hair you just cut. Using the previously cut hair as a guide for length, cut the hair you are holding up.

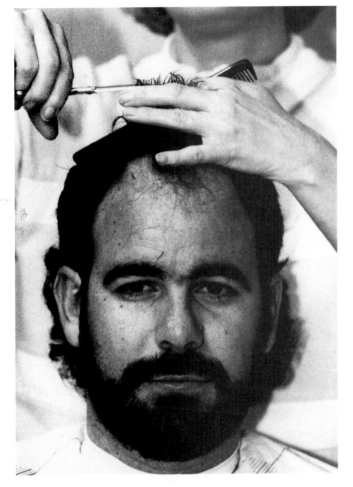

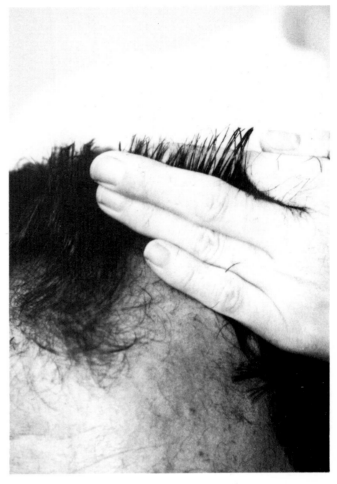

B-3 Continue picking up and cutting horizontal sections of hair until you have cut the entire top. Be sure to always include some previously cut hair in each section to serve as your guide for the length.

B-4 You must now blend the top hair with the side hair. At the front of the side, pick up a finger length of hair that includes some hair from the top and some hair from the side. Hold this hair straight out from the head.

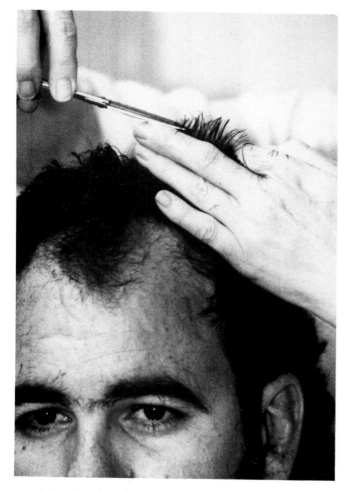

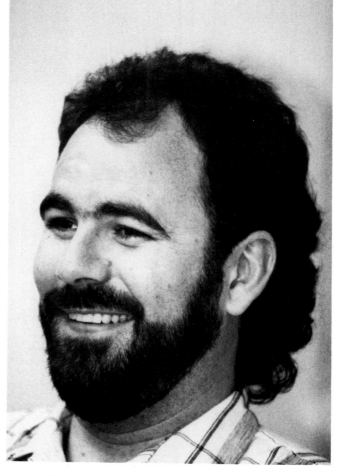

B-5 Cut this hair on an angle from the length of the top hair to the length of the side hair.

Continue parting off and cutting sections of hair that lie along this ridge until you have worked your way to the back.

Repeat this procedure on the other side of the head.

B-6 The top and sides are now complete. The back can be cut following the instructions described in the basic haircut.

Perming thin hair will often make it look fuller. A body wave or curl will hold the hair away from the head and give it more volume.

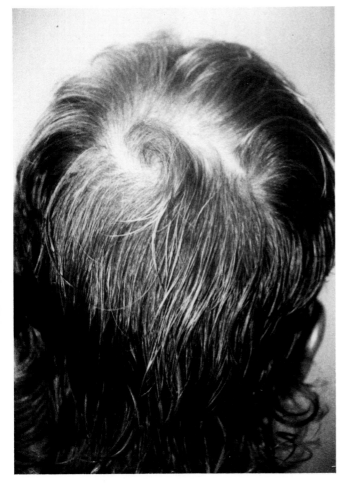

Before Perm

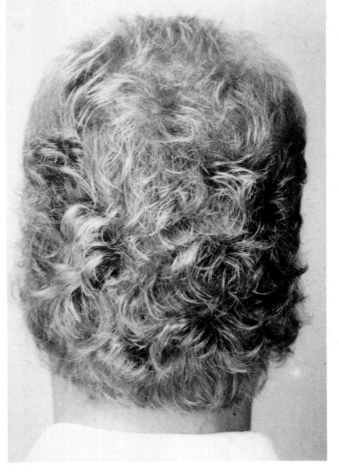

After Perm

BEARD AND MUSTACHE TRIM

Facial hair on men has always been popular. However, an untrimmed beard or mustache looks sloppy and detracts from the overall appearance of the individual. Following these instructions will enable you to maintain a beard and mustache and achieve the best look possible.

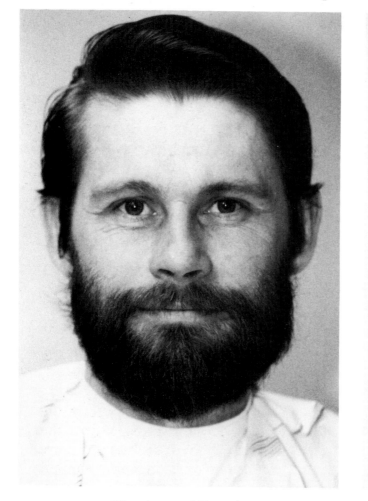

Untrimmed Beard   Trimmed Beard

TRIMMING WITH SCISSORS

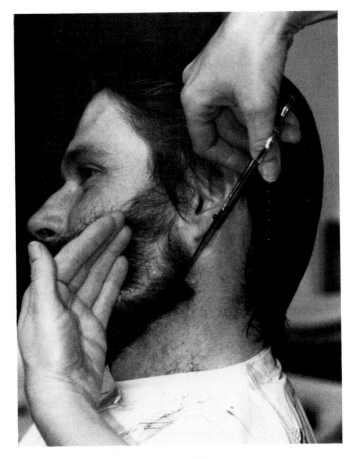

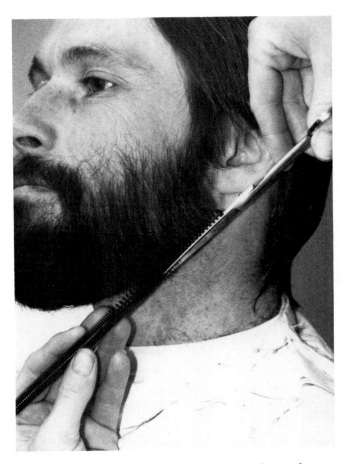

A-1 The jawbone will serve as your guide for getting the bottom of the beard even. If the beard is long, lift it up so that you can see the jawbone line. Beginning below the ear, cut the beard so that the bottom is just below the jawbone. Cut down, following the line of the jawbone until the jawbone curves around to form the chin. At this point, continue cutting down and under the chin. After you have cut under the chin, begin on the other side and cut down, just below the jawline, until you come to the point where you previously stopped cutting.

A-2 Starting on the left side, place the comb along the bottom line of the beard, laying the teeth of the comb flat against the face. Pull the comb away from the face until it is holding the beard up at the length you wish to cut the beard. Be sure that you are holding the comb straight and snip off any hair that is sticking through the teeth of the comb.

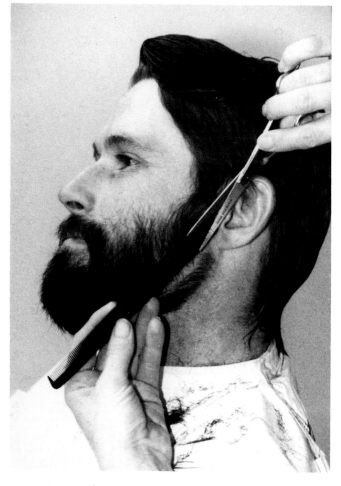

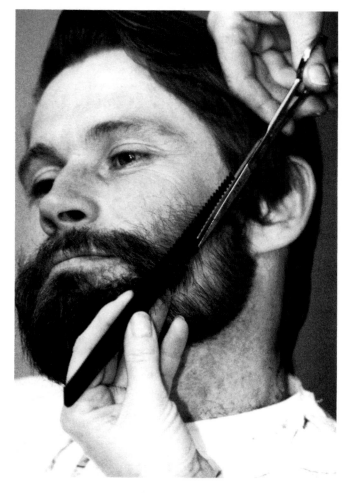

A-3 Place the comb just above the level you just cut. Pull the beard away from the face with the comb, holding it the same distance away from the face as you did on the lower section. Snip off any hair that is sticking out through the teeth of the comb.

A-4 Continue holding out and cutting sections of the beard, always moving up the face.

After you have cut one side, cut the beard covering the chin and other side, using the same technique.

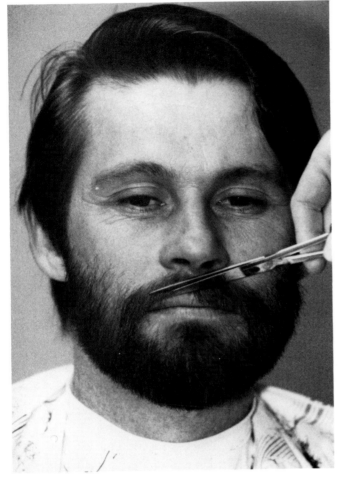

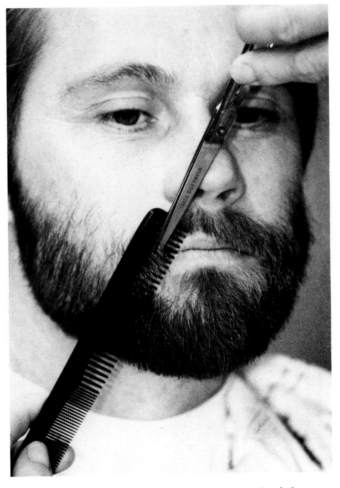

A-5 Beginning in the middle of the mustache, cut it at a level just above the top line of the lip. Remember to use small snips.

A-6 With the comb, lift up the end of the mustache where it grows into the beard. Include with this hair some of the beard that has already been cut. Cut this hair on an angle, blending from the mustache hair to the beard hair.

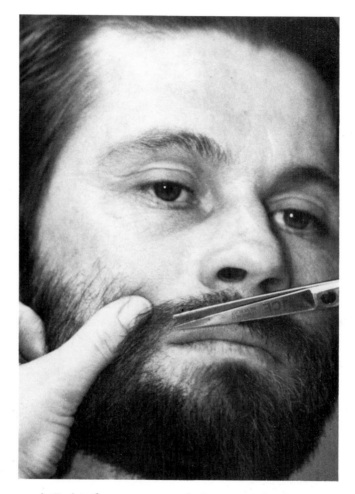

A-7 At the corners of the mouth there will be some hairs that were missed. To find these hairs, pull back on the lip slightly with your thumb. This will allow you to see these hairs and cut them off short.

The beard is now trimmed.

TRIMMING WITH CLIPPERS

A beard may also be trimmed with electric clippers. This method can be fast and easy, but should only be used on beards that are full and thick. Beards that are medium to thin will end up looking too thin when trimmed with clippers.

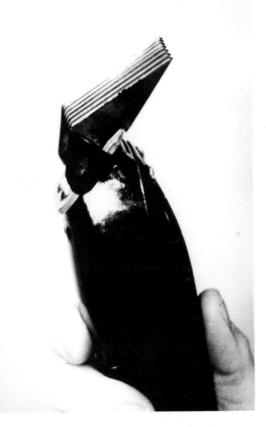

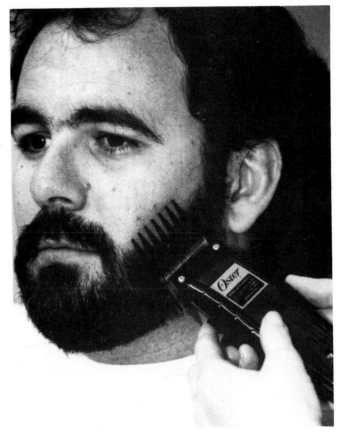

A-1 If the beard you are going to trim has not been trimmed in a long time you will need to establish the bottom line of the beard. To do this, see step A-1 of "Trimming With Scissors."

Clippers come with different sized attachments. Begin with the fitting that has the largest teeth.

A-2 Turn the clippers on. Beginning at the side, run the clippers up through the hair from the jawbone to the top of the beard in a straight, vertical line.

Continue trimming vertical strips of the beard until you have gone over the entire beard. When cutting, always cut up from the bottom moving toward the top.

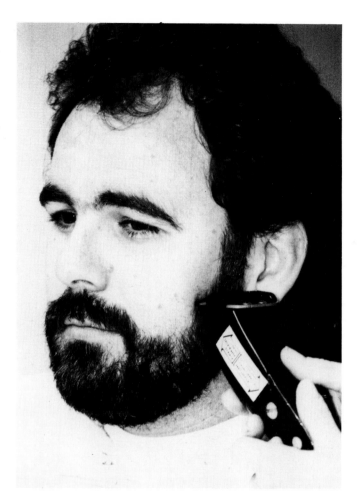

A-3 Remove the large tooth attachment and replace it with the small tooth attachment. The smaller teeth will even up the beard by cutting any long hairs that may have been missed.

Hold the clippers so that the flat part of the teeth point up and the ends of the teeth point towards the beard. This is the opposite way that you held the clippers when using the large tooth attachment.

Beginning at the side, run the clippers down the beard, from the top of the beard to the jawbone, in a straight, vertical line.

Work your way around the face by cutting the beard in vertical strips. Remember to always pull the clippers down while you cut.

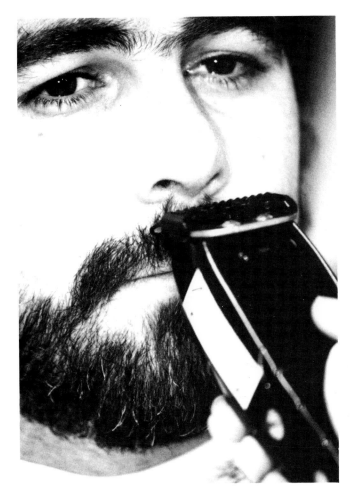

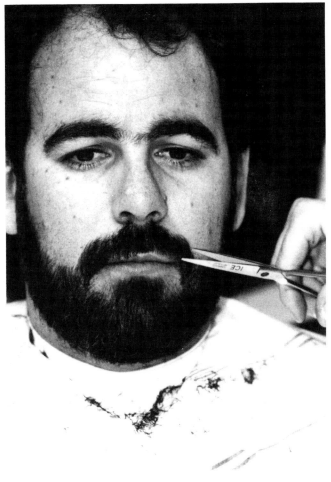

A-4 Pull the clippers down over the mustache.

A-5 With the scissors, cut the mustache at a level just above the top line of the lip. Always use small snips when cutting the mustache.

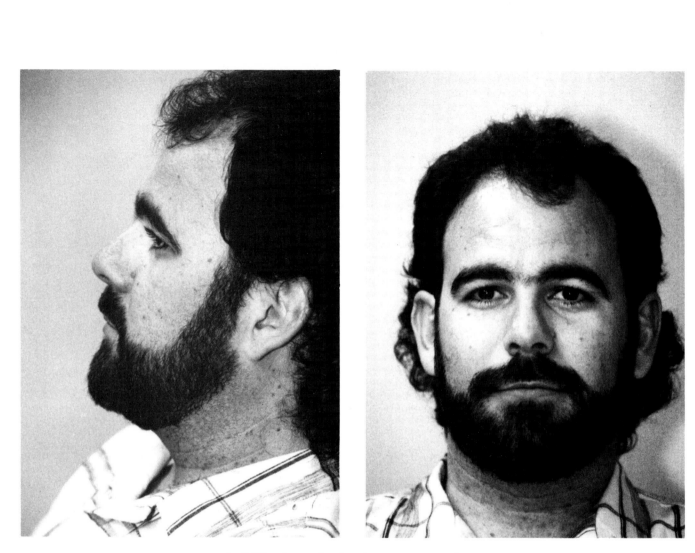

A-6 The beard trim is now complete.

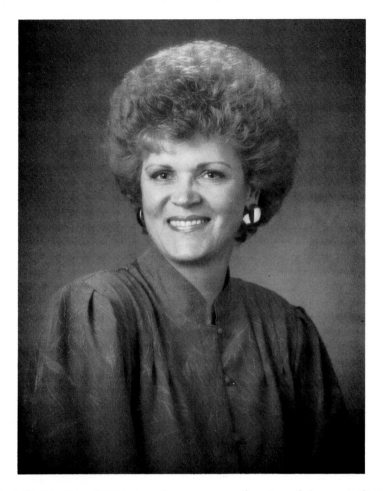

CAROLYN TAYLOR has been a professional hair sytlist for over 25 years, operating a thriving salon in Burley, Idaho. Devoted to her craft, she attends many classes and seminars each year to keep abreast of the latest developments in hair care.

A personable lady who is active in church and civic affairs, Carolyn is known as a woman who can be trusted. This reputation has led many people who are *not* part of her regular clientele to contact her for hair cutting advice.

"I realize that many individuals who are attempting to style hair at home do not understand the basic principles. Consequently, they end up with a bad haircut. As more and more people came to me for advice, or help to repair a poor cut, I determined that there was a definite need for a guide that would demonstrate hair cutting techniques for 'home' stylists. If this guide will help to fill that need, it will be well worth the time and energy expended to complete the project."